AF710164

For People Who Make Love

For People Who Make Love

A DOCTOR'S GUIDE TO SEXUAL HEALTH

JOHN J. SECONDI, M.D.

Preface by Jesse E. Steinfeld, M.D.

Taplinger Publishing Company · New York

This edition published in 1975 by
TAPLINGER PUBLISHING CO., INC.
New York, New York

Copyright © 1974 by John J. Secondi, M.D.
All rights reserved. Printed in the U.S.A.

No part of this book may be reproduced or transmitted in any form or by any means, electronic or mechanical, including photocopy, recording, or any information storage and retrieval system now known or to be invented, without permission in writing from the publishers, except by a reviewer who wishes to quote brief passages in connection with a review written for inclusion in a magazine, newspaper, or broadcast.

Published simultaneously in Canada by
Burns & MacEachern Ltd., Toronto

First published in the United States in 1974 by
Bantam Books, Inc., under the title
For People Who Make Love: A Guide to Sexual Health.

Library of Congress Catalog Card Number: 74-20214

ISBN 0-8008-2965-4

CONTENTS

FOREWORD

This book is for people who make love. It is intended as a means of understanding the diseases caused by germs that have come to live in the sexual parts of the body and are therefore transmitted by sexual contact. A mountain of ignorance smothers the subject of the venereal diseases, and with that ignorance comes fear that prevents people from doing anything about venereal problems. When it is understood that these diseases are subject to the same principles of cause and effect and cure as other diseases, anyone suffering from them can more easily know what to do about them. There is no magic about venereal diseases, and very little mystery any more. The magic is in the lovemaking and is there to stay, and the mystery vanished with the now-easy cures available at every doctor's office. If this book can get you to separate the two and help you take care of yourself, it will be a success.

I have tried to make this book enjoyable reading. A sense of humor separates us from our problems and puts them in a perspective that shows them as they really are: smaller and more manageable than they seemed. You should feel happy when you finish this book because you have been informed how to free a happy subject—sex—from medical inconvenience.

After you read the book through, you can keep it handy for reference when questions arise. Please note that there is a section (Chapter Ten) telling you where to go for help if you don't already know.

Sincere thanks are freely given to several people for their invaluable help to me in writing this book. First there is Ted Bent, author, editor, agent, and friend, who believed in this book before the idea that anyone would listen to information about venereal diseases had made its way into the newspapers, magazines, and television, and who fought a hard and winning struggle to get this book published. Without his unselfish efforts in its behalf, this book simply would never have been.

Second, Dr. James B. Lucas, former assistant chief of the Venereal Disease Branch of the Center for Disease Control (formerly Communicable Diseases Center) in Atlanta, in two full days of personal discussion gave me the benefit of his own expertise in the subject of the venereal diseases. Dr. Lucas was sounding the alarm about the epidemic proportions of venereal diseases years before almost anyone would listen. There are few people, if any, in the world with his knowledge of the subject, and he has been extremely gracious to me. Dr. Lucas is currently serving as dermatologist with the National Institute for Occupational Safety and Health in Cincinnati, Ohio.

A close personal friend, Brobson Lutz, a senior medical student at Tulane Medical School, has done most of the library research for this book. In relaying articles and information to me, his lightning use of the Xerox, the mails, and the telephone can only be referred to as a new art form. Brobson is just becoming an M.D. but already he has established himself as a brilliant original thinker and formidable research scientist in public health, among other fields. The possibilities for his success in the future are boundless. To say that without his research and astute editorial comments this book would have been impossible would be a gross understatement. I look forward to the pleasure of watching his accomplishments multiply.

My staunch ally and critic, Grace Bechtold, executive editor at Bantam Books, has been the very model of a helpful, understanding, and elevating editor. She fused the dual loyalties an editor has for her publishing house and for her author and forged a book that is stronger and smoother and more penetrating for her efforts.

Finally, special thanks go to Dr. Jesse L. Steinfeld, former surgeon-general of the United States Public Health Service, who is currently at the Mayo Clinic. Dr. Steinfeld expressed interest in this project many months ago when it was first mentioned to him and graciously agreed to preface the book with his own overview of the venereal disease problems we are facing today. Dr. Steinfeld brings to his high position an extraordinary intellectual keenness and great personal kindness, not only in executive considerations of his public responsibility, but also in the private prerogative of personal interviews. It is a great honor to have had his encouragement and comments.

John J. Secondi, M.D.

PREFACE

Even today it is extremely difficult for most people, including doctors, to entertain the idea that *nice* people might have a venereal disease. Just a few months ago, a venereal disease epidemiologist approached a young lady in her late teens who had been named as a contact of a patient treated for gonorrhea. The young lady was not too surprised at having been named as a contact, because she was aware that her fiancé had been treated. She was confident, however, that *she* wasn't infected. The reason was that she had been to her family doctor the day before. He had done a microscopic slide smear of a specimen of her vaginal fluid and had given her, as she put it, "a clean bill of health." With some persuasion, the physician agreed to reexamine the girl, making vaginal and rectal cultures instead of just taking a smear. (Smears are *very* inefficient at detecting gonorrhea.) The following day, when the culture plate showed the presence of the gonorrhea organism, he completed the diagnosis of gonorrhea and treated the patient. Friendly questioning revealed that the physician actually had dismissed the thought that she might be infected and had done the smear more to put her mind at ease than for anything else.

The same problem exists with syphilis not being

considered in nice people. It can't be stressed strongly enough that bona fide intimate contacts to infectious syphilis, as well as contacts to gonorrhea and other conditions, need treatment regardless of signs, symptoms, or serology, and regardless of whether they are *nice* people.

One young man noticed a lesion on his penis in mid-October and went to see his physician about it. But his doctor told him that it wasn't anything to worry about. A week later the lesion was still there, and swelling in the groin had developed. At that, the young man went to see his company doctor, who referred him to a dermatologist. The dermatologist referred him to a urologist. The urologist suspected syphilis and referred the patient to a private laboratory. There, finally, a test was made and was found positive.

These are not rare cases. Over the years, the Public Health Service has become aware of many patients with various dermatologic signs of early syphilis who were treated for one thing or another without syphilis even being considered, apparently because the patients were middle-class, well educated, and well dressed.

The reported incidence of syphilis is now over 95,000 cases annually; I would estimate *actual* cases at over 250,000. Gonorrhea is out of control in the United States: we have a national epidemic of major proportions. Reported cases have reached an all-time high, having topped 718,000 cases in fiscal year 1972; and we have evidence to suggest that the actual incidence has passed 2,500,000 cases a year. Syphilis or gonorrhea—one or the other—strikes somebody in this country at a rate of one every 15 seconds.

These diseases are not uncommon in areas and among groups in which they are *least* suspected. Unfortunately, for example, there is a vast unawareness among school authorities of the extent of these diseases; and even when the possibility of venereal disease infection comes to mind, most of us have been conditioned to dismiss it with respect to ourselves or to persons to whom we relate, whether this relationship be familial, social, or professional.

Mainly what people want to know is how they can avoid these diseases and what to do about them if they don't avoid them. I doubt that we're going to do much good if doctors confine their advice to warnings about avoiding exposure. "Exposure" will continue whether doctors warn against it or not.

People need to know such things as the fact that, if coitus is involved, the condom, used properly, will help prevent venereal diseases. With so much frankness in our mass media today about other formerly taboo subjects, it is a mystery to me why we do not see greater reference to this proven venereal disease preventive. And incidentally, the Public Health Service has encountered many people who were under the impression that *coitus* was necessary for VD transmission, and who felt quite secure that if they pursued any kind of sexual activity other than coitus, they would not risk either pregnancy or venereal disease. It isn't so.

Have we lost control? For gonorrhea, the answer is yes; we seem clearly to be losing the battle, if not the war.

We must change our attitudes. By pretending that "nice people" don't get venereal disease, we encourage obliviousness to prevention; second, through our moral indignation toward the "wages of sin" incurred by people who do get venereal diseases, we encourage sick people to delay treatment even if they suspect or are certain that they have a contagious disease; and third, since treatment is delayed through fear or embarrassment of self or others, the spread of these diseases continues unchecked.

I think it is incontrovertible that we are losing control of venereal diseases and other sexual problems because we have not faced up to the realities of modern life. If Americans of all ages will read this book and follow its advice, we will have taken a giant step toward control of these all-too-common, yet easily preventable and curable diseases.

Jesse L. Steinfeld, M.D.

Mayo Clinic, Rochester, Minnesota
Former Surgeon-General of the United States, 1969–1973

Chapter One:
SOME SACRED COWS LAID TO REST

There is a natural human tendency to ignore difficult questions: "just leave it alone and it will go away" is our reaction to any particular annoyance, either consciously or subconsciously. We convince ourselves that nothing is wrong when we know otherwise. We create myths out of half-knowledge that take on the aura of irrefutable and even divine wisdom. As we perpetuate our ignorance and fear, we move farther from solving the original problem.

Nowhere is this habit more true than in our dealings with what have come to be known as "venereal diseases." We have done psych jobs on ourselves singly and collectively. No one on the verge of making love wants to think about the possibility of getting the clap from an opposite number, much less bring up the subject openly. And when you're not making love you certainly don't want to think about VD. Doctors have learned to skirt the subject; although they routinely inquire about bowel habits, spots before the eyes, alcohol consumption, tics, and neuroses, they never think to look for hidden venereal disease. The nation's newspapers, magazines, movies, and television shows have until recently tiptoed around the entire subject of diseases associated with sex with the daintiness of conspiring ballerinas. Social groups, like church organizations and civic clubs, have avoided the subject like the plague, and anyone who dares bring up the matter is immediately branded as—God knows what. The public in general has supported this silence; but although they remain ignorant of the matter, they are certainly not in bliss. The laws of many states are restrictive and require parental consent before treatment of minors for VD. The person, especially the young person, who develops a sore or discharge in private parts is often at a loss for what to do or whom to approach, fearing instant recrimination, even from doctors. For these reasons and for others, people have tended to let things run unchecked, spreading disease to others and worsening their own conditions.

Recently, of course, attempts to reverse these attitudes have had some success. Certainly the term *venereal disease* is being heard frequently everywhere now. *Newsweek* magazine did a cover story on the situation, and other publications have brought the new epidemic of gonorrhea and syphilis out into the open. The Public Broadcasting Corporation put a lengthy and gutsy television show on the air using top name performers and writers to popularize the idea of taking care of VD before it takes care of you. The medical profession is learning to ask questions even when there is no apparent reason to do so, and to change old misconceptions about the sort of people who have the problem. Although venereal disease is not quite fashionable yet, it is certainly getting a lot of (overdue) attention.

Unfortunately there are a lot of deep-seated misconceptions about venereal diseases still generally held by most people. Some wrongheaded ideas about the venereal diseases should be attacked first if we are to distinguish and defeat them.

Even in this "enlightened" world where people realize that there are many ways to have sex and to talk about it other than the narrowly circumscribed ones of the past, people still are reluctant to bring up the possibility of acquiring a disease as a result of having sex. Too few people know or permit themselves to acknowledge the possibility for themselves—or even for others!—that men can get venereal diseases from men, and women from women. Public silence on these subjects still tends to condemn those who stray from the old ways and shame people out of getting medical care when it is needed. But why? It has *always* been common to have oral and anal sex, in addition to penis-vagina intercourse, for men *and* women in every society and social class. When will we pull our ostrich heads out of the sand and face the reality of sex, which has always been more of a smorgasbord than just meat and potatoes? In *all* forms of sex the venereal diseases can be transmitted, and no particular type of sexual activity has a monopoly. If we are to deserve the description of being "enlightened," we should, on the one hand, attack the diseases more vigorously and, on the other hand, leave sex to take care of itself. Nobody's type of sex is "better" or "worse" or more prone to cause disease. Do what you want to do and let others do what they want; get help when you need it and don't raise your eyebrows when somebody else needs medical care for something you don't do. Live and let live; love and let love. This book is for *all* people who make love.

What Is "Venereal Disease"?

The term *venereal disease* or *VD* probably has done more harm to the public than any single germ. There is no such thing as "venereal disease" in the sense of a single disease that comes from venery (lovemaking), as the name seems to indicate. There are a number of different, totally unrelated diseases caused by separate species of contagious agents that are frequently carried in the sexual parts of the body and that together comprise the group of illnesses that can be termed *the venereal diseases*. Some people casually refer to venereal diseases or VD when they mean only syphilis. Other people mean gonorrhea when they say VD. Still others mean both syphilis and gonorrhea by the term *venereal disease*. They are all wrong. Venereal diseases include gonorrhea, syphilis, and a whole range of other diseases that will be thoroughly described in this book, including those due to crab lice, scabies mites, vaginal protozoan and fungal infections, and so on. *A venereal disease is any disease that is transmitted from one person to another in a significant number of people by sexual contact, either by vaginal intercourse, anal intercourse, or oral-genital contact, or by lengthy body-to-body contact.* To call only syphilis or gonorrhea venereal disease is to ignore other important sources of illness arising incidentally from making love.

Always refer specifically to the problem at hand. The term *VD* only clouds the issue and can even lead to panic; the word has taken on a connotation larger than life. If you identify what's bothering you with the correct name, you will realize that the disease in question has a specific cause and a specific treatment program to follow. You will be well on your way to curing the problem and avoiding it in the future. *All the venereal diseases are treatable—completely treatable—if you take care of them early enough.*

What's This About an Epidemic?

When public health experts speak of an epidemic of the venereal diseases, they are referring chiefly to gonorrhea, which has risen in incidence in the past few years to levels that require massive screening and public health measures, rather than the usual one-on-one doctor-to-patient routine that suffices for isolated cases. That's what an epidemic is: a sudden outburst of reported cases of a disease in numbers indicating massive and quick spread of a disease. In epidemics the public health services must go out and look for everyone who might be affected in order to stop the rapid distribution of the disease.

Gonorrhea and Syphilis in Brief

Gonorrhea is a pus-forming disease resulting from certain bacteria (the *gonococci*) that through evolution have learned to live in moist internal crevices of the body called mucous membranes. That means they have preferentially settled in the vagina, the mouth of the womb (the "cervix"), and the egg-bearing tubes (oviducts) of women; the inside of the penis of men; and the throat, mouth, and rectum of both sexes. When the gonococci arrive at one or more of these sites, they multiply. Pus is formed as body cells attack them. Gonorrhea basically does its damage by local destruction, the pockets of pus often scarring the inner tubes of the male and female genital and urinary passages. But gonorrhea germs can spread through the blood to other parts of the body like the joints, the heart, the brain, and the skin. Such spread to other parts of the body is prevented by early and adequate treatment and occurs in only 2 percent of untreated cases.

By contrast, syphilis is a disease caused by a germ that can burrow through the skin—even uninjured skin—and settle in any part of the body, although it too, through evolution, has developed a particular liking for the thin skin of the sexual organs. Syphilis germs (called *spirochetes*) do not cause pus but actually destroy the tissue directly, replacing them with sores and/or scar tissue. Primary syphilis sores are called *chancres* (pronounced SHANG-kers). The disease of syphilis is much more dangerous than gonorrhea because in at least a third of untreated patients with syphilis, terrible complications will ensue years later involving the heart, blood vessels, and brain, causing great deterioration of mental and physical function of the person. At present there has been a rise of syphilis cases in the U.S.A., but not quite to the proportion of gonorrhea cases. Numbers of syphilis cases are measured in the tens of thousands, whereas gonorrhea is commoner and counted by hundreds of thousands, or even millions.

Syphilis and gonorrhea germs make their way through the population separately and only coincidentally turn up in the same person. If you get gonorrhea, you may or may not get syphilis. Some people think that syphilis is a "bad" form of gonorrhea or a complication, which is absolutely not so. Needless to say, the more people you have sex with, the more exposure you get, the greater the risk of getting either or both diseases.

What About the Other Venereal Diseases?

There are a number of other diseases that travel on or in the sexual organs that are easily confused with the two "major" ones, gonorrhea and syphilis. Other germs can cause the same sort of pus discharge and irritation of the gonococci germs of gonorrhea; the symptoms are the same, and you need a doctor to figure out the difference. These other germs are very rare in comparison to the prevalence of the gonococci, however.

There are a number of skin diseases that affect the groin and are transmitted from one person to another that can look like the sores of syphilis. Chief among these are chancroid disease, lymphogranuloma venereum, granuloma inguinale, and herpes simplex virus blisters. These diseases are becoming more common, and you should never leave it to your own discretion whether the sore or rash is "bad" enough to see a doctor about. If it is unusual enough to catch your attention, bring it to the attention of your physician. He will set your mind at ease, either by discovering an innocent cause for your rash, or by giving you treatment for something more serious.

Who Gets Venereal Diseases?

Will people ever believe that VD can come to anyone who has sex, and not just to other, "dirty" people? There are still people—even medical experts—who believe that syphilis is confined to the economically disadvantaged, or to blacks, or to homosexuals, or to "other" groups of one kind or another. The fact is that because of sexual and social mobility nowadays, germs can travel up and down the social ladder many times in a week and multiply very quickly. Rich suburban swingers are just as likely to get the clap as people with smaller bankbooks. Furthermore, the "minor" diseases like chancroid and granuloma inguinale, which were thought to be limited to blacks from tropical areas, are showing up in whites. Crabs and scabies mites, formerly thought to be a sign of uncleanliness, are very common in sexually active, middle-class people. Diseases for which the sexual mode of transmission was previously unknown—like infectious hepatitis from oral-genital contact—are being shown to hit many people via the sexual route. Don't assume for a second that you are "safe" from certain problems just because you are white, or because you live on a farm, or because the bill collector is not knocking at your door.

Why the Epidemic?

There are many theories as to the cause for this or that venereal disease problem. People say that syphilis is on the increase because penicillin no longer is effective. That is absolutely not so. Even after 30 years, penicillin is completely effective against all clinical types and stages of syphilis in relatively small doses.

Some people speak hysterically of the "Asian strain" of gonorrhea acquired during the Vietnam war and imported to this country; the "Asian strain" is supposed to defy penicillin with Oriental tenacity. Again, absolutely not so. After a careful review of all these resistant cases, the United States Public Health Service (USPHS) has put out a new penicillin schedule for treatment of gonorrhea that is highly effective against all strains of gonorrhea now known. So it is not that medicine is losing the battle against the germs. If patients get to the doctor, they can be adequately treated.

There are many experts who feel that one reason the epidemic has developed is that physicians are not reporting their cases of syphilis and gonorrhea to the Public Health Service so that public health workers can track down infected contacts and help them get treatment. There is undoubtedly some truth in that theory. One study from Oregon shows that only about 25 percent of cases of gonorrhea and syphilis are reported by private physicians to the Public Health Service for one reason or another. National figures for reporting are even lower. Gonorrhea cases especially go unreported, since there are so many of them. Many doctors feel they would be swamped by paperwork if they had to report every case, particularly "clap" doctors who see only patients with venereal diseases. However, there seems to be a greater cooperation developing now from private physicians, as they realize the magnitude of the problem we are facing and the need for physicians to work cooperatively with each other, with patients and their contacts, and with public health personnel to fight the problem.

Sometimes The Pill is blamed for it all. There is some truth to this theory, because undoubtedly, with the risk of pregnancy removed, men and women have felt much less reluctance to "risk" the consequences of sex. Since The Pill does nothing to lower the risk of getting a venereal disease, its use adds to the VD rate for many reasons. One effect of use of The Pill is that condoms are not used as often. Since condoms help prevent the spread of venereal diseases as well as prevent conception, their absence makes the VD rates go up.

Homosexuality is blamed for the rise. All of a sudden, America is discovering homosexuals, as though they never existed before. What is really happening is that homosexuals are identifying themselves much more often and with little or no inhibition. It is doubtful that there has been much of a real rise in homosexual activity in America, merely a rise in the reported number of homosexuals coming to medical attention. There has undoubtedly always been a significant component of venereal diseases among homosexuals, as among all sexual types.

Some people blame bisexuality. As a matter of fact, the bisexual male is probably a significant transfer point of gonorrhea and syphilis because he can involve both sexes, penises, vaginas, rectums, and all. There is very little investigative work exploring the statistics of bisexuality.

The common thread among all the contributing factors given above to explain the rise in venereal diseases is that PEOPLE ARE HAVING SEX MORE OFTEN WITH MORE PEOPLE. It is no secret that sexual behavior has changed in the last 10 years. Whereas teen-agers 10 years ago would neck and pet and brag about it, now they screw right away and say nothing of it. Married couples have sex with other mates very casually and often. Some unmarried people, particularly in urban situations, have sex with many people a month. Whether or not you approve of all this sexual activity, that's the way it is, and as doctors and patients we have to realize it and, if problems arise because of increased sexual activity, learn how to deal with them.

The Anonymity of Modern Sex

A few years ago there was a movie with Dustin Hoffman and Mia Farrow called *John and Mary.* The two met at a painfully awkward singles bar and spent the next night and day together, mostly in bed. The film takes us through their 24 hours together and ends as they—finally, offhandedly—get around to telling each other their names.

This plotline is not so far-fetched as it seems. One of the problems in recognizing and treating the venereal diseases is that the person who comes to the attention of the doctor may not know from whom or where he or she got the disease. Anonymous sex is the rule of the day for many people who get venereal diseases. Group sex scenes are fairly common in big cities and many rural communities also. Casual pickups at bars are often forgotten the day after, and no name or telephone number is exchanged. People fly to beach resorts for a week or two and may meet and sleep with several people from all over the world. There are homosexual baths in large cities where men have sexual contacts for a few seconds or even hours without saying a word. Contacts are immediately lost; how could anyone ever retrace such fleeting situations? Therefore, the person who is sexually active with a large number of people, or who has occasional sex with people he can't get in touch with again, must look after himself and take precautions to keep himself healthy. If you get a venereal disease and can get in touch with someone you know or suspect to be at risk, so much the better. But if you don't know where you got whatever is bothering you, take care of yourself.

Morality, Sex, and Disease

Of course the greatest stumbling block in a rational approach to venereal disease—and to many other diseases—has been the confusion in the public mind between sex, sin, and disease. Ever since the Book of Job was first read, men have assumed that disease is a punishment for sin. Venereal disease is assumed to be the classic example of this divine retribution.

The entire science of medicine is based on the refutation of this dangerous superstition. Diseases are acquired because of specific causes that overwhelm the body's natural defenses; in the case of contagious diseases, as venereal diseases all are, germs are obtained during sex that take hold and cause an infection locally in or on the sexual parts. If the doctor or the patient is to deal with this fact effectively, he must remove himself from the realm of breast-beating and guilt and think about cause, effect, and cure. *We must learn to treat venereal disease as simply another disease.* After all, venereal diseases can be acquired in ways other than lovemaking; doctors, for instance, have had to risk getting syphilis merely by touching and examining their syphilitic patients. And syphilis can be transmitted innocently via shared needles, blood transfusions, and pregnancy. The germs concerned will travel any way they can travel. There is nothing inherently sexual about them; it is merely that they have found an evolutionary niche in the genital areas, for the most part, but not exclusively, and certainly not as a divine retribution for sex. The universe works on perfect rules of cause and effect that we imperfect mortals understand only partially. But one thing should be clear to all: when certain forces build to such strength that the normal integrity of the human body is compromised, disease occurs. This is true for the common cold, tuberculosis, and venereal diseases alike. God does not interfere with the perfect logic of his universe to punish individuals with disease. Some of the biggest real sinners are in perfect health. Diseases are subject to the same rigid laws of cause and effect, and it is up to us as disease-ridden people to interpret those laws as best we can and, working through them, lessen the effects of illness. It is no more a sin to have venereal disease than it is a sin to have tuberculosis.

Whatever your views about sex, you are entitled to them. This book deliberately avoids making any "moral" judgment on any sexual practice whatsoever. Disease has nothing to do with morality; it is a problem to be attacked by a rational set of tested procedures. Learn to attack the disease, and to separate it in your own mind from sex itself. One does not give up eating all apples because there was a worm in one.

Self-diagnosis and Self-treatment

There are a lot of subtle points of difference between the forms of venereal diseases that are best left to physicians to pinpoint and cure. Syphilis, for instance, can mimic a number of lesser diseases, only some of which are venereal. The nonphysician who happens to have a penicillin bottle in the medicine cabinet left over from a sore throat a year ago is doing himself and everyone else a great disservice by swallowing a few tablets and letting it go at that. This procedure is sadly a lot more common than you would guess. There are very few diseases that the sufferer can diagnose and treat without a doctor's help. The purpose of this book is to help you identify problems so that you can begin to understand them and differentiate between them. Modern society wants to know about diseases in real terms, and not in medical mumbo jumbo. The truth is always fascinating, especially in medicine. But this book is not intended for you to use to start a self-help VD clinic. Learn to spot problems on yourself and others, and refer to this book when you need to, but get to a doctor if something turns up.

No Symptoms Does Not Mean No Problems

Unfortunately, something will not always seem wrong if you have a venereal disease. You can have the germ and give it to others and risk severe complications in later life without noticing any symptoms at first. Syphilis very often goes unnoticed, especially chancres of the vagina and rectum, which no one sees without medical equipment. Gonorrhea in the vast majority of women is not noticed because of the many hidden recesses of the female genital anatomy. *This means that if you have sex frequently with different people, you are going to have to check on your venereal disease status regularly even if nothing seems wrong.* Otherwise you stand a great risk of slipping into the tertiary phase of syphilis and/or incurring the complications of gonorrhea, both of which can be disastrous. A person who has frequent sex with different people should have a blood test for syphilis at least once a year, and preferably twice a year. A woman who has sex with different people should have routine cultures of her genitals annually along with her Pap smear test for cancer. These tests are cheap. In some cities, syphilis blood tests are given free at public VD health clinics or by social groups like gymnasiums or public baths and spas. Only if you keep a tab on your blood test for syphilis can you be sure to avoid its late-blooming complications. If you have sex only with your husband or wife and he or she doesn't take a lot of trips out of town, don't bother to have this regular checkup more than every few years. It is the exposure to different people, not the frequency of sex with the same person, that increases the risk of infection.

Vaccines, Preventive Pills, and Other Pipe Dreams

Every now then you see a longing in the press for a vaccine against venereal disease. There are no vaccines or shots you can take to prevent a single one of the many venereal diseases, much less all of them. There are difficult problems in developing specific blood tests for gonorrhea, and even greater ones in the research for a gonorrhea vaccine. Any preventive shots or oral doses to be taken like the polio vaccine is taken now, for instance, are a long way off. And since we are dealing with such diverse problems as crabs, scabies mites, hepatitis, and several skin infections of the groin, there is probably never going to be any all-inclusive "vaccine" to take to avert all these problems. If you have sex with different people a lot, you are simply going to have to be on the lookout.

About (Not) Acquiring Immunity

There is no immunity to any venereal disease. You can get syphilis, gonorrhea, crabs, scabies, lymphogranuloma venereum, chancroid, granuloma inguinale, herpes simplex eruptions, *Trichomonas vaginalis, Monilia* fungus, and so on again and again and again. You must cure each case thoroughly each time you get it, and you must cure everybody with whom you have sex if you are to get rid of whatever you have. And then you must keep on the lookout for a new problem in the future. There will be no "relapses" if the treatment has been thorough and effective. If you play doctor, however, you are likely to give yourself an inadequate dose of drugs and the disease will calm down for a while before flaring up again. (Infectious hepatitis is not primarily a venereal disease and does bestow some immunity.)

Let Calm Prevail

It can be very disconcerting to discover that you, the cleanest and nicest person since Joan of Arc, have crab lice. *Lice!* Or pus on your underwear. Or an ugly sore on the skin of your genitals. You may get a sinking feeling in your stomach and begin to reassess your whole world view. Don't panic! These things have been around for centuries and are very common even among your dearest friends and in the very best of circles. There are a lot of famous names highly revered in the history books and idolized in the newspapers who have had worse venereal problems than you; you just don't know about them. Stay calm. Realize that no disease is pleasant, and that venereal diseases are no worse than most other infectious diseases and a good deal less bothersome than most. A broken knee causes you a great deal more difficulty. We are fortunate to live in an age when diseases that terrified other times are handled in five minutes in an outpatient clinic and cured in two days of antibiotic treatment! Until this century, syphilis was the cause of insanity in millions of people, and nothing could be done about it once those unfortunate people had caught the germ. Now all cases of syphilis are accountable to penicillin and many other drugs. Period. Just like that. Most other venereal diseases are as easily treated. Get yourself to a doctor and consider how lucky you are by comparison. In most cases, you won't even have to refrain from sex.

A General Approach to Follow

Most of what you read about the venereal disease spectrum is in terms of epidemiology, which is the study of disease as it affects the population as a whole. These statistics cite millions with gonorrhea, thousands with syphilis, and so on. All of this is of little value to you as an individual, other than alerting you to the risk *you* run. Either *you* have something, or you don't. It is all or nothing with the individual, not 35 percent. The entire approach of this book is to help *you,* one single human being, deal with problems you may have or think you may have, and decide what to do about them. Don't worry about the thousands in Pedula with such-and-such. Worry about yourself and those you come in contact with. That way you will be doing what you should be doing for the health of yourself and those you care about, and you will be contributing to reducing those large statistics and percentages as a whole.

Chapter Two:
COMMON INFECTIOUS ITCHES AND DISCHARGES

Introduction

When a woman goes to her doctor and complains of a vaginal itch or discharge, as many millions of women do, the most common diagnosis made is *not* gonorrhea or syphilis. Often there is some chemical or fabric irritation of the vulva, or some hormonal, steroid, contraceptive, or drug reaction. A most common cause of vaginal discharge and itch, however, is infection, usually with certain yeast or protozoan organisms. All of these disturbing forces just named cause roughly the same disruption, damaging the normal surfaces of the vagina and producing an irritation, itch, and reactive white blood cell discharge. In most cases, symptoms such as these give no absolute clue to their origin. *All* cases must be diagnosed and treated by a doctor.

There are some purists, both experts and inexperts, who object to including the topics in this chapter under the heading *venereal disease* at all, on the grounds that these infections are not *known* to be *exclusively* transmitted by lovemaking. They argue that since the term *VD* has had such a stigma attached to it, it would be well to avoid applying that term to the millions of people who get the diseases discussed in this chapter, and to leave that term to the classic pair, gonorrhea and syphilis, and maybe to a couple of others. Thus would be spared a great deal of "anguish." It seems to me that excluding these yeast and protozoan infections from our discussions of VD would be wrong for several reasons. First, *these diseases are the most common venereally transmitted diseases in the world!* The evidence that these infections are spread frequently through sexual contact has been substantiated largely in the last 10 years, and both doctors and laymen alike need to be educated to this fact. When a disease is spread through sexual contact, treatment that does not get to both sexual partners is no treatment at all. And whereas syphilis affects people in this country in the thousands and gonorrhea in the hundreds of thousands, millions of people (mostly women) suffer from trichomonal or monilial infections, sometimes for years. A tormenting itch is "anguish" enough no matter what we commentators call it. The point is to get the person to the doctor, and to get the doctor to treat all the sexual partners involved. It should be noted that for the most part the diseases mentioned in this chapter cause inflammations and discomfort localized to the area of the genitals. There are no systemic complications or severe long-range derangements as in syphilis and gonorrhea. Nevertheless, if left untreated, these diseases can cause years of suffering.

If we are ever to get rid of the idea that there is a stigma about getting sick, we had better stop slinking away from sexual diseases or labeling them with inaccurate preciosities. If you have a Protozoa in your vagina or penis making you miserable that can easily be transferred to your man or woman, you have a venereal disease. Suffering is cured by correct diagnosis and therapy, not by calling the disease by another name.

Trichomoniasis: the "Trick," Its Itch and Discharge

Trichomonas vaginalis is a microscopic one-celled organism that parasitizes the human genitourinary system. It has a rather poetic ring to its name, a perfect trochaic tetrameter; to pronounce it, accent every other syllable, beginning with the first. The "ch" is pronounced hard, as in "trick." In fact, it has been nicknamed just that, doubtless by some gynecologist wag somewhere. The disease it causes is called trichomoniasis, or *trik-o-mo-NI-ah-sis*. The symptoms of intense itching and bothersome discharge that so often affect women with the disease are neither poetic nor humorous, however.

There are no reliable statistics of the incidence of this disease, but it is estimated that at least 2.5 million women between the ages of 20 and 50 in the U.S. are infected with *Trichomonas* Protozoa; perhaps as many as 10 percent of all women harbor the Protozoa in their vulva, but not all get symptoms from them. There are many unanswered questions about the disease. There is a great variance in symptoms and discomfort produced in different people. Since the disease is venereal, it can be assumed that there are as many men with *Trichomonas* infection as women; yet women complain of vaginal itch and discharge much more than men are known to suffer from penile discomfort. Some men and women seem to have an immunity: although trichomonads can be cultured from them, they never have any symptoms. Some women seem very resistant to infection, and others very vulnerable. Some women are easily cured, and others may have recurrences for 30 years.

It is known that the trichomonal organism can live in the vagina as a harmless bystander, and that by itself it can cause no more damage than, say, the germs in your throat. However, if something happens to alter the natural resistance of the vaginal surface, the Protozoa can burrow in and cause the itch. White blood cells then come to the site of inflammation and are sloughed off eventually as the unpleasant discharge. This white cell debris is called *leukorrhea.* The delicate balance of the female vaginal wall depends on correct hormonal regulation, favorable vaginal acid-alkaline environment, and, perhaps, nervous system stimuli. Oral contraceptives alter the natural hormonal ratios and also directly radically change the acidity and configuration of the vaginal covering; it seems clear from numerous studies that *women on oral contraceptives have a higher incidence of trichomonal infection.* There is also a correlation between trichomonal infection and menstrual disturbances from other causes.

Men seem not to get symptoms as much, perhaps because the natural irrigation of the entire outflow tract by urine several times a day clears the Protozoa away naturally. The female anatomy does not have this natural flushing mechanism over all the surfaces exposed to infection.

There are no clear-cut conclusions to be found in the medical literature about correlation of the risk of getting *Trichomonas* infection and socioeconomic status, race, or circumcision. The incidence is higher in women of the childbearing group, presumably because with increased sexual activity the risk of acquiring the Protozoa goes up. Transmission seems to be largely sexual; there are no reported cases of toilet seat or shared undergarment transfer in the literature as yet. There is an increased incidence of gonorrhea among people with trichomonal infection, and vice versa. Whether this is due to the coincidence of both organisms preferring the same parts of the anatomy, or whether there is some cause-and-effect relationship is not known. Having more sexual partners increases the risk of multiple infections with any of these agents.

Symptoms

When a person—let us say a woman, since women are troubled so much more by the trichomonads than are men—develops symptoms of trichomoniasis, does she get some clue that this problem is due to this particular Protozoa and not to gonorrhea or some allergic reaction or hormonal-menstrual problem? No. Many of these organisms send out the same initial signals. There is an incubation period of from 4 to 20 days after acquiring the Protozoa. Then, a vaginal discharge *may* begin. Many women will get no discharge at all, or a quantity small enough to ignore. In the "typical" patient, however, there is a copious, foamy, greenish yellow vaginal discharge accompanied by soreness and itching of the vulva and the skin in the thighs. The discharge may smell bad. It is common to have had some discomfort at recent sexual intercourse. Pain on urination and unaccustomed frequency of urination are mentioned, but less commonly.

In some women the onset of these symptoms may be sudden and dramatic, and the patient can almost pinpoint for her doctor the moment it began. The discharge may be profuse, with extreme soreness and swelling of the vulva; intercourse may be difficult or impossible, and life in general may suddenly become very miserable. Needless to say, this set of symptoms cannot go long without medical attention. (Frequently this condition arises a few weeks after a honeymoon, when a virgin bride first sleeps with her experienced husband.) In other women, infection may be chronic, getting worse after occasional menstrual periods.

Men are generally symptomless, but after careful questioning may remember itching and discomfort inside the penis, with perhaps a slight wetness at the end of the penis for a few days. These symptoms often disappear spontaneously, whereas in women, once symptoms are noticed they almost never go away by themselves.

Diagnosis

Although there may be an infected male for every infected woman, the diagnosis is usually made in women, since women usually need to seek medical attention. A thorough pelvic examination is made. Often the physician sees a characteristic "strawberry" mottled appearance of the vaginal wall, indicating trichomonal irritation. Slides are made of the discharge and examined within a few minutes under a microscope; the diagnosis is usually made right then, on the first visit. In addition, cultures are made for trichomonads and for monilial fungus (see below) and for gonorrhea. The physician will probably do a Pap smear (a simple smear of cervical drainage to look for signs of cancer) at the same time, complete the pelvic examination, and draw blood for a syphilis blood test, just in case.

In men with a discharge severe enough to require a doctor's attention, the first disease to be looked for is, of course, gonorrhea, but cultures and slides for *Trichomonas* should be obtained when the gonorrhea test is negative. The physician may want to examine and culture the men whose women came first to the doctor and had trichomonal infection diagnosed.

Treatment

Since 1960 the treatment of trichomoniasis of the genital tract of both sexes has been made easy by a drug known as metronidazole (Flagyl®). This drug is effective when given orally two or three times a day for 10 days; results are probably no better when vaginal medicine is given in conjunction. The sexual partner(s) MUST be treated simultaneously or the effort is wasted. There is no need to refrain from sex with the PREVIOUS sex partner, but wait till the week is up before tackling anyone new. You need not worry about undergarments, bed sheets, or anything else.

Moniliasis ("Candidiasis," or "Thrush")

The yeast *Candida albicans* is to the Protozoa *Trichomonas vaginalis* as Tweedledee is to Tweedledum. They are inseparably linked in every doctor's mind because of their common symptomatology; they are clinically difficult to distinguish, but a good microscope or culture always tells the truth.

As with *Trichomonas,* presence of the *Candida* yeast in the vagina does not ensure that symptoms will occur. Active cases of candidiasis require some factor to tip the scales in favor of an overgrowth of the yeast; classically, the use of antibiotics for other diseases has been known to change the chemical environment so that fungi such as *Candida* flourish. Diabetics have a distinctly higher rate of moniliasis, as the glucose in the urine provides food for the yeast. Taking oral contraceptive pills and other steroid drugs alters the vaginal pH (acidity) enough to help the *Candida* yeast. Pregnancy also increases the risk. Whatever the cause, *Candida albicans* yeast is now the number one cause of vaginal discharge and itch.

Symptoms

There really isn't a dime's worth of difference between these symptoms and those of trichomoniasis—to the patient. Intense irritation, itching, and a discharge are the chief complaints. The doctor's questioning may elicit some nuances, however. In moniliasis, the discharge is whitish and cheesy-thick. The discharge may tend to adhere to the vulva or vagina. The vulva is often red from irritation and tends to swell more than in trichomoniasis. Onset may vary, again, from spectacularly quick to insidiously slow. Without treatment in mild to moderate cases there can be successive recurrences and remissions for years. Severe cases cannot go unnoticed.

In men, symptoms are much less bothersome, as is the case with trichomoniasis. There may be a low-grade urethral inflammation, with little or no discharge. The most common symptom in men is itching due to an irritation of the foreskin of the penis.

Diagnosis

For women, complete pelvic exams are done in which slides and cultures are made for both *Trichomonas* and *Candida*. In men, cultures are attempted from the tip of the penis. Diagnosis is usually made in the office at time of examination with a slide or two under the microscope.

Therapy

There are a number of antibiotics used in pessary (vaginal suppository) form for women. Local application of gentian violet for several weeks to the affected areas is still an effective treatment but requires several thorough applications by the physician. For men, there has until recently been little therapy available other than an excessive oral fluid intake to flush the yeast away, but amphotericin solutions through the urethra are indicated when infection is not removed by simple fluid therapy. Various creams containing nystatin are effective. At present, therapy for candidiasis is not quite as neat as for trichomoniasis, and since these diseases tend to hang around quietly for many years waiting for a chance to flare up again, follow-up visits to the doctor and follow-up cultures are often suggested.

Hemophilus vaginalis and Obscure Causes of Irritation

Hemophilis vaginalis is a bacterium known to exist in normal and in irritated vaginal vaults. Recently attempts have been made to determine whether it and similar, previously ignored bacteria could account for some of the unexplained vaginal discharges and itches. Not all labs are equipped to culture for these rarer, less delineated types of vaginal and urethral irritation.

In cases where doctors have eliminated gonorrhea, trichomoniasis, and candidiasis as causes for itching and/or discharge, the diagnosis may be pinned on a bacterial agent such as *Hemophilus,* and a "broad-spectrum" antibiotic may be prescribed that is effective against a wide range of such bacteria. "Nonspecific urethritis" in the male corresponds to these nonspecific discharges and itches in the female. (See the section on nonspecific urethritis at the end of the chapter on gonorrhea.) These exceptions, alas, point out that not all is yet certain in medicine. You should understand why your doctor may have to pin an unsatisfying, nonspecific diagnosis on you and treat you practically, perhaps in some way not even suggested in this chapter.

Pinworms

Hemophilis vaginalis is a tiny one-celled bacterium, *Trichomonas* a large one-celled protozoan, and *Candida albicans* a large one-celled yeast. Pinworms, of course, are visible, sophisticated, multicellular, organized animals. They are placed in this chapter because it now seems that pinworms are a cause of vaginal irritation, itch, and discharge in a number of adult women. Until recently, most physicians assumed that only infants or little girls could have pinworm irritation spread to the vaginal area from the anus and rectum. However, a very new study reported to me by Dr. James Lucas at the USPHS in Atlanta shows that even in college girls, a small percentage of those with vaginal complaints had pinworms demonstrable. The risk of transmission by sexual contact is unknown, but may be estimated to be very slight. However, we mention this topic so that physicians and patients alike think to look in cases of vaginal discomfort unexplained by the more common diseases.

Summary

The organisms in this chapter cause localized irritation inflammation, pus formation and discharge, and the symptoms of itching, burning, and general discomfort particularly in the vagina but also in the penis. The diseases they cause are the most common venereal diseases in the world. The first three organisms—*Trichomonas, Candida,* and *Hemophilus*—are very large one-celled microorganisms many times the size of bacteria. As such they may cause allergic reactions locally in the sites of infection that aggravate the suffering of the host. Pinworms are tiny parasitic animals on a much higher scale in the zoological hierarchy, but can cause much the same sort of suffering in women. All of these diseases are treatable with the proper agents. Complications are rare, although in certain people allergic hyperreactions may occur. Once treated, the patient does not build up an immunity and runs the risk of reacquiring the organisms if they are reencountered. Men who have *Trichomonas, Candida,* or *Hemophilus* infections in their urethras usually carry very few organisms and, lacking symptoms, do not suspect they have the disease. In these cases, they are the unknowing reservoirs of the organisms that spread the disease. Women generally do feel symptoms of itching, burning, and some discharge but may be inclined to ignore the problem as "normal" for women. Unless the suffering woman gets to the doctor and both she and her current sexual partner(s) are treated, medication is futile.

Chapter Three:

CRABS, LICE, AND MITES

Lice are as intertwined with history and language as they are in body hair. The English vernacular has colorful monuments to the tenacity of these little creatures, although word origins are often forgotten. For instance, calling a person a "louse" or "lousy" used to mean just what the words say. And nit pickers were originally people who waste a lot of time searching out lice eggs (nits) one by one instead of finding a broad solution to the problem.

Having lice used to mean being "unclean." If you were dirty, you would presumably acquire lice; if you developed a louse infestation, you were admitting to being dirty. Unfortunately, this attitude is still common and tends to prevent "nice" people from seeking proper treatment. As with any disease in this book, lice are no respecters of persons or privilege. These days cheerleaders and Miss America contestants can get them; the tweedy and the funky; heterosexuals and homosexuals; physician and patient alike. Lice thrive on physical contact, not on dirty habits.

There are three kinds of lice that live off humans:

crab, body, and head lice. All of these are transferred from one host to another by direct physical contact.

Crab Lice

Description

Of the three kinds of lice—crab, body, and hair—crab lice are the most common in America, and the least dangerous. They are also the only kind that live exclusively on sexual parts of the body and are considered to have an inherently "venereal" means of spreading. They are not known to carry any diseases beyond the nuisance of their own infestation. Crab lice (*Phthirus pubis*) are universally called "crabs" because, under a magnifying glass, they look like crabs. They are visible to the naked eye, but only in a good light, and are compared to "dandruff flakes" or "freckles," depending on the metaphorical bent of the observer. Once you know what they look like, they are unmistakable the next time around.

Life-style

Crabs live mostly on the pubic hair of the crotch, often on the armpit and stomach hair, and occasionally on the hairs of the thigh and the trunk, on a hairy male. The reason they have come to prefer these sexual areas is an evolutionary coincidence. The size of pubic hairs and the distance between individual pubic hairs are different from those of other body hairs. Crabs' legs just happen to be the right size to grab hold of two pubic hairs and dig in. Occasionally they are sideswiped by an oncoming eyebrow or beard and are forced to take up residence where they are not really comfortable. That is why eyelashes, beards, and sideburns occasionally acquire crabs.

Once crabs grab hold of their two hairy anchors, they feed on the skin itself and do not move to adjacent surfaces such as clothing willingly. They lay their eggs on the bases of the hairs. Adult crabs live about a month and lay about 50 eggs in a lifetime. The eggs are one-fourth the size of the adults and are securely glued to the hairs. Eggs can be seen as tiny crooks or bends in the hair that are, on closer inspection, translucent granules not easily removed. When the eggs mature, they migrate to new areas on the same person. Because of the limited area to be covered, no more than a few dozen crabs are found on a single person; but even one crab is enough to cause itching and discomfort.

Contracting the Crabs

If you have any sort of physical contact with the private parts of a person with crabs, you will get them too. Crabs are not eager to leave one person for another, but if the contact is hot, wet, and long, they inevitably do. Occasionally crabs are left behind on sheets, towels, and underwear, and any object that has been closely applied to the body of the infested host. Crabs are an occupational hazard of emergency room nurses and physicians, who have all of the risks and none of the pleasures of close contact. Although no studies have been done, it is thought that public rest room toilets have a rare incidence of harboring cast-off crabs that (for a short while) survive to find a new host. These risks of indirect transfer are very, very slight, however.

The adult crab cannot live more than three days without a host; newly laid eggs have a grace period of two weeks before they die, as adults, of starvation. So the only significant means of spread is person to person.

Diagnosis

Usually you don't discover the crabs, they find you. Out of the blue you will itch sharply and suddenly and scratch with abandon, perhaps unconsciously. You may even jump out of your chair the first time. The itch will persist and demand closer investigation. It is confined to the pubic hair and the genital-anal region, usually. The itch comes and goes, and does NOT wake you up at night. Crabs may be inhibited from multiplying rapidly by normal use of soap and water, but they never go away by themselves no matter how much washing you do.

To look for them, go to natural sunlight or use an incandescent light. Adult crabs are on the skin surface; eggs are found on the hair shafts. Any "freckle" that starts moving is immediately suspect: crabs are frequently the color and size of small freckles. If they have just hatched, they may look pale gray and translucent, especially on black skin. Nits—lice eggs—are much more numerous and are best seen if you move the hairs back and forth. Even after a long infestation, you will find 10 or 20 at the most. After you've found one, you've made the diagnosis; stop nit picking and move on to therapy.

Treatment

Don't panic! It doesn't mean you're not a nice person. Don't shave your pubic hairs: when the stubs grow back, that itch will be 10 times worse than that of the crabs. Use one of the following:

A-200 Pyrinate®. This is a pleasant, semioily liquid with a rather enjoyable smell. No prescription is needed. With your hands spread enough of the liquid to cover the following areas: all your pubic hair, all the hair on your stomach, chest, nipples, and under your arms, and any hair on your back and shoulders. If your arms and legs are densely hairy, cover them too. There is no need to use any of the lotion on your head. Leave the A-200 on about 15 minutes, then comb away all the nits, take a hot shower, and throw the comb away.

Cuprex®. This is the old standby, but it is now totally obsolete, except for masochists. It stings like crazy and can actually give you a rash. If you think you need to suffer even more from your "transgression," by all means use Cuprex®. Use it exactly like the A-200.

Kwell®. Another coal oil derivative, 1 percent gamma benzene hexachloride, this comes in three forms: a cream, a lotion, and a shampoo. In some drugstores it can be bought without a prescription, but in most cases you will have to see a doctor. The cream and lotion are used exactly alike: First take a hot soapy shower, then dry yourself thoroughly. Then apply the cream or lotion over every inch of skin from the neck down. Don't miss a single square inch. The film seems to "disappear," but leave it on for 24 hours and forget about it. *Do not wash* during those 24 hours. Then take another shower and be sure to use all freshly washed clothes, as with other treatments. (This treatment will also kill the mites of scabies.)

The Kwell® shampoo is the easiest treatment of all. Lather it into all the hair mentioned in the section on A-200 above, and wash hard for at least four minutes. Wash the shampoo out and comb the nit shells out.

In all cases, wash your underwear, sheets, towels,

and pants used in the period when you were infested. Hot water temperatures kill any stray eggs. Unless you have had prolonged sex on the blankets or bedspreads, you can avoid a large dry-cleaning bill. Crabs are not highly motile; they cannot "jump" to the bedspread or sweaters or to anything else.

With all of these remedies, one careful application should do the job. Everyone with whom you have slept or had other direct personal contact should get the same treatment *at the same time.* Warn household members who may be at risk to make an examination of themselves.

You should tell everybody with whom you have recently slept, matter-of-factly, so that he or she can be treated promptly. Don't try to figure out who gave it to whom; that too is nit picking. After treatment, refrain from sex for 15 minutes. Any further self-denial is unnecessary after a thorough treatment. There is no need to go to a physician for a case of crabs unless you have a complication such as an infected scratch mark or an unrelated but sexually acquired disease.

Try to avoid getting paranoid over these creatures; they are absolutely unassociated with any serious disease that other kinds of lice carry and can be gotten rid of in 15 minutes with a minimum of discomfort and a hearty shrug. The next time you itch, forget it; it's your imagination. If the itch comes back again, look. Don't sit for hours under a strong light waiting for freckles to move across your belly. Some people who sleep around a lot check themselves every night routinely; that sort of thing is ridiculous. The incidence of crabs is on the rise, but the situation is still uncommon. Fortunately, once the crabs are gone, so is the itch.

Body Lice

Although the body louse—or "cootie"—is a first cousin of the crab, its life-style, method of extermination, and danger are altogether different. Body lice feed on all parts of the body, not just the genital areas. But recent trends in communal living, communal sex, and sexual mobility have made sexual transfer an important method of spread, and that is why we include body lice in a discussion of "venereal" diseases.

Life-style

Body lice—simply called "lice" in most casual discussions—feed off the body several times a day and more often at night, but they do not live all day long on the body surface itself. They live and lay their eggs in the clothing or bed linens of the affected person, concentrating in safe crannies like seams and hems, and move to the body surface only to feed. These activities mean that at any given time only a few lice will be found on the body itself, in light infestations, but the clothing will be loaded with adults and nits, posing a threat to the entire household.

Body lice are more prolific than crab lice, and a healthy female may lay 275 to 300 eggs over a 20- to 30-day life-span. A British woman named H. P. Hudson estimated in 1917 that one female could give rise to 112,778 grandchildren in 48 days. There is a report of 25,000 lice being found in the clothing of one individual. Body lice are more likely to be found on persons who don't change clothing frequently.

Recent reports have indicated a surprising rise in incidence of body lice among young people who prefer casual, communal life-styles, sharing beds and clothes. Communal living is made to order for body lice. When sexual contact is made with someone from outside a commune, a few eggs may go with that person and spread the disease to others with noncommunal habits. Once again, washing with soap and water can only slow down, not cure, the infestation. Therefore, if we may extrapolate from recent literature, medical practitioners and sexually active people old or young, gray flannel suit or levis, should be aware of the very slight, but growing, risk of getting body lice.

Diagnosis

Body lice are the same size as crabs, but are noticeably less round and somewhat thinner and longer. Under a magnifying glass the adults are easily distinguished from those of crabs if the body and clothing distribution haven't tipped you off already.

The symptom is a generalized itch caused by louse saliva injected into the bite site. Whereas the itch of crabs is strictly confined to the groin, that of body lice shifts from one spot to another like foursomes of tennis players and is more severe. This almost incessant itch *is* enough to wake you up at night. Scratching is so intense that large scratch marks may be developed over the body.

To find body lice, first look in your groin to see whether you have the crabs. Next, check the back of your neck and your head hair to determine whether you have head lice. Then, inspect your underwear carefully. Look specially in the seams. Lice are the same color and general size as crabs. Eggs are pale gray and smaller than the adults and appear as gritty granules in the seams in large numbers.

Treatment

Getting rid of body lice is a complicated matter and requires the coordination of a physician to eliminate the risks to the household and to watch out for diseases that body lice carry. Treatment does not center on the body, but on the clothing and other sources of reinfection. In addition to using the Kwell® lotion for 24 hours all over your body, you must destroy heavily infested clothing and bedding and disinfest your home with an insecticide. (Since FDA declarations on pesticides are now in flux, your doctor will have to recommend an approved one to you.) Personal items, including bedspreads, blankets, coats, sweaters, and so on, must be steamed clean and treated with insecticide. If anyone in your household has lice, everyone may be presumed to have them.

You must dispose of, or send to the cleaners, all the affected fabric items before you use the Kwell®. Then, on the same day, have everyone in the household take a hot soapy shower, dry thoroughly, and apply Kwell® over the body, not missing one square inch. The lotion will seem to "disappear," but it is there; leave it on 24 hours, and then wash it off. When you wash it off, you must have all clean clothing, bed linens, and other fabrics to use.

Since sexual contact has become a major mode of spread of body lice, any bodily contact with a lousy person may be presumed to guarantee acquisition of at least one louse. Therefore, if you have body lice, you should refrain from sexual contact with anyone outside your immediate household for several days after you use the Kwell®. You should not bring anyone into your household for two weeks after you disinfest all the linens. Needless to say, depending on the size of your household and your linen supply, this may have to be modified. That is why a doctor is needed to advise.

It is to be noted that body lice carry such extremely serious epidemic diseases as typhus, relapsing fever, and trench fever. Although these diseases are rare in the U.S. today, they are by no means unheard of. It is the body louse, through epidemic typhus, that killed off Napoleon's troops even more than the winter and the Russians. Don't toy with these creatures; be sure to see your physician for guidance.

Head Lice

Head lice are the same size (a small freckle) and shape (long and thin) and have the same life expectancy as body lice, but have adapted themselves to nearly exclusive residence in the hair of the human head. (In Australia, sideburns are known as "lice ladders" for this reason.) In the past women were thought to be more commonly at risk because of longer hair. Such suppositions no longer hold in this age of the peacock.

Life-style

Lice live near the roots of the hairs and on the long shafts of the hairs. They lay their eggs on the hairshaft near the skin; as the hair grows, the nits are carried outward on the shaft; so you can tell how old the infestation is by judging the number of nits and their distance from the skin. Hair lice and especially nits are present by the hundreds or thousands, but surprisingly most victims have no idea that their itch is the result of being parasitized. They are aware only of an intense itching sensation and more often than not develop irritated red areas, scabs, and crusts from scratch marks before going to a doctor for help.

What kind of contact spreads head lice? The chief mode is still crowd situations: dormitory living, gym classes, schoolrooms, group sex, sharing of athletic supplies and linens, borrowing someone else's brush and comb, and so on. (Mothers are forever telling their children not to borrow combs, although they may have forgotten exactly why: this is the reason.) Head lice are very, very rare and still mostly found in specialized group situations: the GI haircut is basically a mass defense against head lice. As things loosen up, cases of sexually transferred head lice will undoubtedly be recorded.

Diagnosis

Head lice are so happy on the head they don't spread to beards or pubic areas. Therefore, you develop an intense itch on the scalp, and nowhere else. As it is impossible to look for nits and lice on your own head without driving yourself crazy, go to a doctor if you have a severe itch and/or flaky crusts on the head or the nape of your neck. (The adults and nits look like those of other lice, should you spot one.) Be warned: cases of head lice are often misdiagnosed, most frequently as a "rash" or "impetigo" or "eczema."

Treatment

Your doctor will probably treat you with Kwell® shampoo. You should apply the shampoo generously, scrub for 10 minutes, rinse, apply, scrub, and rinse again. You will need to steam-clean or dry-clean any neck scarves, hats, or other head articles that might have picked up a stray louse. Your doctor will also want to inspect and treat all members of your household or dormitory and eradicate incidental eggs in hats, towels, and pillowcases by steam cleaning or an insecticide. Brushes and combs should be washed with the Kwell® shampoo also.

Repeat your shampoo treatment 24 hours later; make sure all your household members get simultaneous treatment. Reinfestation is more treacherous with head lice than with the other forms because the lice are so numerous.

The Mites of Scabies, or "The Itch"

In every chronical from the Old Testament to the present there is at least one footnote paying tribute to the persistence of the mite that burrows in the top of the skin to cause scabies. James I of England declared that "none but kings and princes should have 'the itch,' for the sensation of scratching is so delightful." Whether or not the British royal family suffers from scabies is doubtful, but unfortunately since World War II the mite has been surfacing in all segments of the population again after a period of quiescence.

If the itching of crabs and lice is a nuisance, the itch of scabies is a torment that drives strong men to tears. In addition to direct irritation on the skin surface, the mite (*Sarcoptes scabiei*) provokes in the body an allergic reaction to the microscopic fecal pellets it leaves behind, so that antibodies and chemicals are produced in the bloodstream that increase the itching sensation many times over.

Life-style

Mites are much smaller than lice, perhaps 10 times smaller than the "freckle" we use to describe crabs. Since it is so small and since it burrows into the skin and does not stay on top, the mite is almost never seen at all, even when a clear diagnosis is made. The pregnant female digs into the skin and makes burrows that are described as grayish black streaks at the most a quarter of an inch long. Obviously these lines are hard to find. Since most Americans wash as compulsively as Lady Macbeth anyway, the number of parasites and their marks will be kept down.

After the adult lays the eggs just below the surface of the skin, the eggs hatch in three to five days and the new mites migrate above after three weeks to mate and burrow again. By penetrating the skin, each mite leaves a tiny blister called a "papule" or "vesicle." These vesicles are clear, translucent, or fluid-filled blisters only the size of a straight-pin head and are easily seen in a good light, occurring in groups on the body. Often these areas become red from unconscious scratching before they are recognized.

In the early stages of a first attack there is itching limited to the site of the burrow and the vesicles. Before one is aware, eggs, larvae, and occasionally adults are transferred under the fingernails by scratching to other parts of the body. Then the itch begins to "spread" to other locales. The mite chooses the most sensitive skin it can find. All thin and loose skin is quickly settled in. That explains the preference found for the penis; the testicles; the vulva; the nipples of both sexes; the armpits; the thin skin of the elbow and the side obverse to the elbow; the ankles; the instep of the feet; and the hands, especially at the web of the fingers. And if *any* scabies mites are present, signs are almost *always* found on the web of the fingers on the hand and on the sides and backs of the fingers.

Contracting Scabies

To get scabies you have to have intimate personal contact with an infested person. Although older discussions emphasize the risks in group situations like the army, public schools, and so on, it is now realized that sexual contact is an important route of transference. The new sexual mobility of Americans allows these parasites to enter the wealthiest and humblest of homes in rapid alternation. Emergency room personnel are exceptionally vulnerable because of close contact with so many patients. If you do get scabies from sexual transmission, chances are the itching will start at the genitals and spread to other parts of the body, unlike the crabs, which stay put in the crotch.

Dogs and other domestic animals have their own species of mite that causes "the mange," but such mites are usually not interested in humans. However, there are clearly documented cases in which the human variety of the mite has been acquired from the family pet causing an epidemic of scratching and itching in the whole family. (Mites are *not* anything like fleas—they are much smaller and do not jump around.)

Diagnosis

Modern washing habits have altered the characteristic pattern of black burrow streaks, papules, and red scratch marks that used to be so apparent in the infested person. Washing with ordinary soap and water limits, but never cures, the disease. Since the adult mite is so much smaller than the adult crab, it is rarely seen even by a competent physician. The diagnosis is made by finding at least a few characteristic lesions and by the history and distribution of the severe itch.

The victim begins to scratch at the site of original implantation of the eggs or adult, spreading the eggs with his fingernails. One will probably itch for a few days or more before noticing the vesicles. Then the itch gets worse and the vesicles spread. In a few weeks the allergic reaction ("acquired hypersensitivity") begins and the unfortunate host begins to scratch—or, rather, to gouge—himself all over the body, even where mites do not go. Nothing else matters: grown men, resplendent in Brooks Brothers suits, are reduced to rubbing their backsides on doorframes with ruthless intensity, like African elephants. The itching is unbearable and *characteristically* wakes the victim before dawn.

All of this has several side effects that are as important as the primary disease itself. The severe scratching leaves frequent bloody scabs and secondary infections by bacteria. The patient becomes unstrung and is so demoralized and nervous he is good for nothing else; he cannot sleep at night or work in the day.

The scratching and scabs that give the disease its name may disguise the problem as a severe eczema or impetigo, or even a "nervous condition." Misdiagnoses are common, especially since the telltale burrows and blisters are hard to find. Contagious "eczema" had better be attended to immediately, as it is likely to be scabies.

Sexual contact plays an important part especially because of the proclivity of the mite for the thin skin of the body. All the erotic zones are designed to be just that sensitive. It is not unusual for the itch to begin in this genital area and be mistaken at first for anal itching from pinworms; or crabs; or a skin rash from contact with offensive or allergenic materials. Your doctor will not think of scabies right off the bat; so if you have spotted something suspicious, point it out to him.

Treatment

Despite the awfulness of the itch and the difficulty in identifying the parasitic cause, once the diagnosis is made, the cure is simple and quick. Kwell® lotion (1 percent gamma benzene hexachloride) but NOT the shampoo, has been successful for many years. Take a hot soapy shower. Then carefully apply a generous amount to every inch of your body below the jawline. Don't forget anything—the chest, the back, the nipples, the underarms, the forearms, between the fingers, the fingernails, inside the hollow of the navel, all around the genitals, the anus, the cleft between the buttocks, all areas of the ankles, and between the toes. If you miss the tiniest spot, you will pay the consequences. Leave the solution on for a full 24 hours; don't even wash your hands. Change your bedclothes and wash them, along with your underwear, towels, and shirts. Then forget it. There is no need to do anything to your blankets or upholstery. The risk from indirect spread via clothing is nil. One dermatologist reports that during World War II six hundred Argentinian soldiers with scabies were cured by a single dose of Kwell® lotion for each man for 24 hours without requiring even a change of clothes. Nevertheless, for the best treatment you should wash your clothes.

Of course it is your obligation to see that all members of your household are examined and treated if infested. Everyone you have had sex with for the duration of your itch should be informed and examined too. If you find out that you have had sex with a person infested with scabies, take the 24-hour Kwell® lotion treatment as a preventive measure. Even though you may not even get mites from that person, taking the treatment will reduce the risk to zero.

Although the lotion kills the mites in a day, it does not cure the itching immediately. The bumps disappear within a very few days (usually two or three), but the allergic reaction persists, for days or even weeks, diminishing steadily and gradually to nothing. If you take the treatment, be confident that it is completely effective; you can be sure you do not have the disease any more if the red marks, burrows, and blisters go away, even if the itch persists for a while. It will go away in a month, by the latest.

One further consolation is that scabies mites do not carry other diseases, as body lice do, and that the Kwell® treatment will kill crabs and any other lice you may have picked up. Because of the difficulty in making the diagnosis and the necessity for a prescription for Kwell®, you will probably have to see a doctor about scabies.

Chapter Four:

GONORRHEA (THE CLAP, GC)

Introduction

In what has got to be the silliest medical experiment on record, in the eighteenth century a man named John Hunter infected himself deliberately with the pus of a man with gonorrhea in order to prove that gonorrhea was an infectious disease, distinct from syphilis. He was right, but unfortunately the man coincidentally had syphilis too; so John Hunter eventually died of syphilis and gonorrhea, and the whole great issue of what was what in venereal disease was clouded for over a hundred years. One has the impulse to say "It served him right," except you aren't supposed to say that sort of thing about Great Men of Science.

In the intervening years, gonorrhea has, far more than syphilis, affected millions of people, and until the age of penicillin it was a terribly debilitating disease, especially in group situations like armies, which often lost 20 or 30 percent of their men to sick bay because of the clap. Then penicillin was discovered and overnight gonorrhea, even more than most other infectious diseases, became a "minor" problem.

Well, 25 years later, gonorrhea is the number one reportable infectious disease in the U.S. today. It is the main reason this book is being written. *Over two million people will develop gonorrhea in this country this year, and many of them will not know it unless they look for it.* When they say we're in an epidemic of it, they're not kidding. Why is this? What is *the clap?* In this age of antibiotics, why should an infectious disease be making such a comeback? Along with all the bad jokes, there are a lot of rumors circulating blaming this or that; so perhaps the first thing we should do is define it and erase some of the half-truths you have heard.

Gonorrhea is a specific disease resulting from infection by the "gonococcus" bacteria, or more properly *Neisseria gonorrhoeae*. John Hunter's mistake notwithstanding, it is NOT the first stage of syphilis or any other disease and has nothing to do with syphilis, which is caused by another distinct set of germs. Both simply settle in the same parts of the anatomy, as cars and buses both populate the New Jersey Turnpike. The word *gonorrhea* means a discharge in the gonads, or genital organs; in other words, pus forms from the bacteria somewhere in your private parts and eventually drains out. The gonococcus is very hard to grow in the lab, but it does very well in all wet, warm, mucous-lined surfaces in the body, particularly in the snug harbors of the male and female organs that deal with reproduction and urination (the *genitourinary* tract), the moist areas of the crotch around the vagina and/or anus, and the throat, the mouth, and the rectum.

The recent rise in gonorrhea is attributable NOT to resistance of the gonococcus to drugs, NOT to rumored killer strains from Vietnam, nor from any trend other than one: people are screwing more often and with more different people in very casual ways, without checking up on the possibility of disease. That's it, pure and simple. Dr. James B. Lucas, an infectious disease expert with the Public Health Service, told me that if everybody would simply choose one sexual mate and stick with him or her for six months, most of the gonococcus germs would die off and the entire problem would disappear. There are some problems in diagnosis and therapy; but these are minor ones, no greater than for any other contagious disease. The real threat of gonorrhea is that you can have sex with several people and distribute the germs without even knowing you had them all along. This is especially true of women, who usually have no symptoms at all. (See below.) Increased sexual activity is here to stay, and it's not our job to comment on it. What we must do is learn to move quicker than the bugs do.

Sources and Risks

It would be nice if you could point at one cause and one cure and one prevention for the clap, but these are as diverse as sexual practices themselves. You're almost sure to get it if you're a bisexual U.S. serviceman in Thailand who pops antibiotic pills every now and then at his own whim. You're pretty safe if you're a nun in a convent in Idaho. Read on.

How do you get the clap? For the most part, from direct, lengthy close contact with the genitals of someone who has it. The germ is fragile and requires a good deal of heat and moisture to survive. *You can also get it from the throat or rectum of someone who has it there*. You cannot get it from short kisses or from shaking hands or from sheets or discarded underwear. There *is* reason to believe that if someone wipes off a gonorrheal discharge on a towel, hangs it up, and walks away, and you should run in at that instant and wipe it over your genitals, you can get the infection. The risk of this is, obviously, very, very slim.

If you have sex with an infected person, do you automatically get the clap? No. There are studies that show risk factors. An uninfected woman who has intercourse with an infected man is much more likely to get the germs in the first place; the odds are better than 50-50. Because of the different anatomies, an uninfected man who has intercourse with an infected woman can shed the germs more easily and thus has only a 1-in-5 chance of retaining the germs and becoming infected. The whole nature of infection requires not only the germ, but also a receptive temperature and acidity-alkalinity balance, a stable environment, and so on. In men, germs are often washed away by the normal flow of urine and do not linger, whereas in women, the normal urine flow does not reach all the significant parts to carry germs away.

Because of the complicated sexual and reproductive functions of the female anatomy, there are many more structural recesses and surfaces than in the more simple male anatomy. This provides more places for foreign bodies and germs to hide, and it has been statistically determined that germs can lodge in the female sexual organs in greater numbers and go completely unnoticed more often than in the male. This means that the "reservoir" of gonococci is in women. This does not mean that more women have the clap than men: obviously a women has to get the germ from a man. However, 90 percent of women who are infected because of their natural anatomy feel absolutely no symptoms, or no symptoms bothersome enough to seek help for. This means that many women acquire the germs and the destructive damage of the disease in such a way as never to be conscious of it; they have it until some late complication shows up. In this way, they can pass it unwittingly to men, whereas men, because of their simpler and more direct anatomy, are much more likely to have painful symptoms, go to a doctor, and get cured right away. Often the only way a woman knows she has gonorrhea is to be told by a man to whom she gave it.

Despite the common thought that the gonococci are easily maintained in the female sexual tract, there are other reservoirs that have been overlooked until recently. For instance, NOT all men who get gonococcal infection of the urethra (the penis's urine and sperm tube) have such severe symptoms that they go to doctors. Ten to twenty percent of infected men, like most women, may have no symptoms at any time and don't reach medical attention. Therefore, they also may spread the disease without knowing it. In addition, men who have been diagnosed for the clap and treated are pronounced "cured" after urethral cultures are found to be negative, but a very small percentage of these may harbor disease organisms farther back in their sexual glands (like the prostate) without knowing it and can massage these germs by intercourse into their sexual partners.

Two other moorings of the clap also overlooked until lately are the throat and the rectum, in both heterosexual women and homosexual men. The practice of fellatio (oral-genital sex) was never even mentioned in doctors' offices. The musical *Hair* has changed all that. Fellatio is a common heterosexual and homosexual practice. Several studies have confirmed that sore throats, fever, and tonsillitis are not infrequently caused by gonococcal invasion of the throat. Furthermore, the throat may harbor these germs and serve as a source of infection without the person's ever having any symptoms. You cannot transmit these germs from mere kissing, however.

The rectum is also a very common reservoir of gonorrhea, although it hasn't been talked about much. In one study of heterosexual women in Norfolk, Dr. Harry Pariser demonstrated that fully 40 percent of women with gonorrhea had gonorrhea in the rectum, and 20 percent of those had gonorrhea in the rectum alone, and not in the vagina! The latter group may be presumed to have had rectal intercourse, whereas many of the others may have spread gonorrhea from their vaginas to their rectums passively, with faulty toilet habits or a runny discharge.

The incidence of rectal gonorrhea in homosexual men is even higher. In a New Orleans study, a group of acknowledged homosexuals were given rectal cultures, whether or not they complained of venereal problems. Nineteen percent of those without venereal complaints and 41 percent of those who were worried about gonorrhea had positive rectal cultures. This means that in both sexes rectal gonorrhea can frequently go completely unnoticed while serving as an excellent source of infection for others.

You undoubtedly come into contact with one or more of these sexual sites or you wouldn't be reading this book; so let us describe the symptoms and what you should do about them. Remember two things: First, in many diseases you can be loaded with bacteria and not feel a thing. Second, there are very few specific symptoms in medicine. There are a hundred causes for a vaginal discharge and itch, for instance. Don't jump to conclusions in any case, but don't ignore the problem: see a doctor.

Symptoms and Lack of Them

Inflammation of the Vagina and Urinary Tracts of Both Sexes (Vaginitis and Urethritis)

The incubation period—the time between getting the germ and showing symptoms—is two to five days. This figure applies more to men than to women because 9 out of 10 infected women get no symptoms at all. In symptomatic men or women, within a day or two of exposure to the germs, the urethra becomes itchy and uncomfortable in a vague way. (Of course both sexes have *urethras:* the urethra carries urine from the bladder to the outside.) After another 24 hours, there is a clear-cut "burning sensation" during urination, and the penis or vagina may discharge cloudy drops involuntarily into the underclothes. Frank pus usually develops, but may not. Most men will seek treatment at this stage because of the pus and pain, which can be intense. Women may feel nothing or may have a slight discharge and itching that may not seem serious. Other disorders in women—fungal infections, menstrual problems, changes in vaginal acidity caused by taking The Pill—can simulate the itching, discharge, and discomfort of gonorrhea. If a clap discharge does occur in the woman, it is classically thick, smelly, dirty yellow, and looks clearly like pus; but it may be thinner and more greenish than yellow. Thick, curdy, lumpy discharges that stick to the vaginal walls are probably due to fungus. (See the index for the sections appropriate to these disorders.) In men, pus discharges are thinner but otherwise like the above.

Rectal Symptoms

Rectal clap—the "poop"—also has many guises. After rectal intercourse there may be discomfort anyway; so abnormal symptoms are often hard to discern. With rectal gonorrhea, there may be a slight discomfort accentuated before and during bowel movements. There may be a discharge, thin or with pus. Stools may be thinner or diarrheal. There may be a feeling of fullness in the rectum that simulates a necessity for a bowel movement. There may be systemic symptoms in severe cases, like fever and body aches, but this is rare. In most cases there is just a vague, squirmy discomfort or, most commonly, NO symptom at all. The incubation period is the same as for symptoms in the urinary system.

Sore Throat

Pharyngitis (sore throat) may develop several days after oral sex and may exactly resemble, both to the patient *and* to the doctor, "strep throat," a term that refers only to the sore throat caused by the *Streptococcus* organism, not by the gonococcus. Doctors almost never think of gonorrhea in the mouth in either women or men patients, but they must now begin to think of it every time they see a sore throat. It takes a different culture medium from the one used for *Streptococcus* to grow out and thus prove the existence of the gonococcus germ in a patient. If you find it hard to tell you own doctor to culture for the gonococcus, find a doctor you can talk to. Unless a special culture is made, you'll never know.

In some cases of gonococcal sore throat, the soreness is explosive and cannot be ignored. You will see a doctor right away. In many cases there may be only a transient sore throat or no symptoms at all. You should see a doctor about all severe sore throats you may incur, because there are serious complications to both gonococcal and streptococcal pharyngitis if they go untreated. You should also go to the doctor if you suspect that you may be carrying gonococcal germs in your throat without symptoms. Routine throat cultures are not called for every time you have oral sex or have a minor pain in your throat.

Summary

Gonococci cannot penetrate skin, as the spirochete germs of syphilis do, and therefore have to make their way along the wet linings we have talked about. During a heated sexual exchange the germs can swim around in that effluvium of passionate sweat that sticks to both bodies and travel to these sites of infection.

If you turn up with ANY of these symptoms, or if you suspect that you carry the germs without symptoms, you MUST go to the doctor. Gonorrhea germs linger in the penis and vagina and outer parts of the sexual-urinary tract for months, and you can pass the germs on to many people indirectly during those lingering months. After several months you may no longer be infectious to others, but the germs can thrive in deeper structures inside you and cause severe secondary complications of the clap, perhaps even after you stop being infectious.

Complications

Women

In women, fully 20 percent of untreated patients go on to severe abdominal spread of the germs, involving the *uterus* (womb), oviducts ("tubes"), and ovaries (egg-bearing gonads). These complications are lumped together under the semislang term "PID," or pelvic inflammatory disease, which may be agonizingly apparent or misleadingly silent, but which in either case almost certainly results in reduced fertility or sterility. (Some, but not all, unexplained childless marriages are due to PID in the woman.) What happens is that the gonococcus swims back up the vagina and through the womb to the tubes and ovaries themselves. Here they form pus and eventually scar tissue, just as pus wounds form scars after they drain. Such scarring obliterates the passageway of the tubes, while gonococci spread to the abdominal cavity and form pus there. Obliterating the tubes and/or destroying the ovaries through pus and scar formation can silently cause sterility. Spreading pus into the abdominal cavity causes symptoms of an "acute abdomen" exactly like those of appendicitis. Often the very first sign of gonorrhea in the woman is detected in the emergency room, when the sufferer shows up with "appendicitis": nausea, vomiting, fever, and agonizing pain in the belly. At this stage antibiotics can help but eventually total surgical hysterectomy may be necessary to control pain, which means sterility and dependency on oral female hormones. Needless to say, PID carries a significant mortality rate.

Men

In men, the classic complication is scar formation inside the penis around the urethra, resulting in thinner and thinner streams of urine, severe pain, and finally obliteration of the passageway. This complication is rare today because symptomatic men will see a doctor and get cured with antibiotic therapy before this stage is reached. Nowadays the most dangerous complications are those that involve the hidden recesses of the male reproductive tract where the bugs can cause slow, chronic infection and destruction without arousing much attention from the host. The tough, fibrous maze of the prostate gland, which plays a supporting role in the drama of ejaculation, makes a natural hideout for the gonococcus. Acute prostatitis—inflammation of the prostate gland—can cause pelvic pain, fever, frequent urination, and occasionally painful retention of urine. Chronic prostatitis can linger for months, getting worse with each sexual manipulation. Symptoms include aching in the groin, early-morning clear urethral discharge, and excessive seminal discharge during intercourse; or the symptoms can be systemic, including general sluggishness and a low-grade fever, without any symptoms localized in the groin. Chronic prostatitis is hard to diagnose and hard to eradicate, but it should not be forgotten if any of these symptoms occur.

The third most common male complication is epididymitis, or inflammation of the sperm-carrying bridge in the testicles. The *epididymis* (Ep-e-DID-e-mis) is the tubular structure that connects the sperm-producing testicles with the urethra. The gonococcus in these cases is thought to travel back through the prostate to the epididymis, causing severe pain, tenderness, and swelling in the testicles and groin, and fever. This condition is not rare and should not be trifled with; if it is in both testicles, it will almost surely cause sterility.

Generalized Complications Common to Both Sexes

In untreated cases of both sexes there are several extremely severe complications that are frequently misdiagnosed: the gonococcus can spread through the blood to cause skin infections, arthritis, heart infections, and meningitis (spinal and brain infections). Few doctors think seriously about gonococcal causations for these diseases, and indeed they are rare. Nevertheless, 2 to 3 percent of untreated clap patients—women three times as often as men—will develop arthritis and arthralgias—joint inflammation and joint pains—within a few months of first getting the gonococcal bacteria; and about half that number will get meningitis and heart infections, both of which are among the most life-threatening emergencies on hospital wards.

Disseminated infection, that is, infection seeded from the original genital site through the bloodstream to other parts of the body, is much more common in women because so many have an unrecognized primary genitourinary infection. The spread of infection occurs more frequently during pregnancy, or during menstruation in nonpregnant women.

Arthritis caused by blood-borne gonococci does not look any different from bacterial arthritis caused by any other organism. The joints are red, swollen, painful, and hot. They hurt more while actively moving or being passively moved. Chills and fever may or may not accompany the arthritis. Usually involved are the knees, wrists, small joints of the hands, ankles, and elbows. These symptoms may be great or slight, and the signs of pain and fever may be missing.

When germs flow through the blood—in a condition known as "bacteremia"—they may seed other organs of the body. A few skin lesions may erupt that begin as tiny red, raised areas and evolve through chickenpox stages to large pus centers with or without hemorrhage. Large blisters, often hemorrhagic, may occur. This condition may be benign; that is, the lesions may be easily treated and unaccompanied by any other symptoms or problems. On the other hand, cardiac symptoms may result if the heart valves and muscles are also seeded with gonococci. Chills, high fever, severe discomfort, chest pain, and a feeling of palpitation of the heart may be present, and the doctor may detect heart murmurs on examination. It is not known how many "rheumatic heart disease" cases are diagnosed today that are really classic gonococcal arthritis and carditis. The diagnosis of rheumatic heart disease has been fashionable for some time, whereas that of gonococcal heart disease is not.

Meningitis, or inflammation of the lining of the spinal cord and brain, can also be caused by blood-borne gonococci and results in a morbid state of high fever, delirium, and neurological symptoms. Obviously any patient this ill will come to the attention of a doctor; it is the doctor's duty to be on the lookout for gonococcal disease and not meningococcal germs in a patient with a suspicious arthralgia accompanying the meningitis.

For the patient's sake it should be reasserted that these severe complications occur in *less than 1 percent of untreated people*. In *treated* patients they are unheard of.

Diagnosis

How does the doctor make positive diagnoses of all these entities? The whole field is a chessboard of endless possibilities, but various authorities, guided by the Center for Disease Control (CDC) in Atlanta, which oversees the national attack on every infectious disease from bubonic plague to loa loa, suggest the following:

Any woman who complains of a vaginal discharge or any symptom vaguely referable to sexual activity should see a doctor at once. The doctor should culture the vagina for all the possibilities—the clap, fungal infections, and so on—and give a thorough pelvic exam, perhaps combining it with a now-routine vaginal Pap smear test for cancer cells. For the clap, separate culture specimens should be obtained from the vagina (at the cervix) AND from the anal canal. If the doctor doesn't take a rectal culture and you know he should, tell him. To be sure of cure, this procedure should be repeated weekly for the next two weeks. Of course, tests for syphilis and other venereal diseases should be done at the same time, since these venereal birds often flock together.

In men who complain of symptoms, an attempt may be made to make a slide of any urethral discharge for examination under a microscope. If the result is positive for gonococcus, treatment should begin at once and the patient told to come back in a week for a culture to see if he is cured.

Culturing the rectum is an often-overlooked procedure. If the patient has a good relationship with the doctor and comes in complaining of rectal problems that may be venereal, the culture and the diagnosis can be promptly made. Doctors should remember that some of the most virile, prominent athletes and public figures in the world are homosexual. If the doctor cultures only those who are "effeminate," he will ill serve the cause of health. The best thing to do is to culture the rectum of men and women in whom venereal disease is suspected. Period. Especially when cultures are negative for the vagina or penis. Once the procedure becomes routine, it is never forgotten, value judgments are unnecessary, and no one is offended. Once the diagnosis is made, treatment is the same no matter how many orifices the patient has been employing for sexual gratification.

Throats should be cultured for gonococcus in any patient with a known exposure to an infected person, in any patient with venereal complaints, and in every patient with a sore throat.

In men or women with suspected systemic complications of gonorrhea, blood cultures must be taken. Infected joints should be cultured for all the various causative bacteria, including gonococcus. In meningitis, spinal taps should include cultures for gonococcus if there is the slightest hint of arthritis or gonorrhea in the history. Suspicious skin lesions require direct culture and blood culture, as does rapidly progressing eye reddening or pain (*conjunctivitis*). In these cases it is up to the doctor to be on the alert, as the patient either will not think of the venereal connection or will be in no shape to help.

These culture techniques are not new or radical. The recent advances in growing these fastidious gonococcal organisms in a laboratory are merely refinements in packaging the culture media. The real problem is getting the doctor to think of doing the culture in the first place. How many physicians are receptive to the idea of doing routine rectal cultures for gonococci in women? Yet this is essential for the health of 40 percent of all women exposed to gonorrhea, and for the population as a whole. The doctor must learn to err on the side of overculturing and must make rectal and throat cultures for gonococci a part of his daily routine. Furthermore, the doctor must suspect these germs even if a garden club type walks in with a vaginal itch, or if a professional hockey player complains of a poopy feeling in his rectum. The patient must lead the doctor in many cases. Think of the possibility yourself and mention it. It's your disease, and your cure. Don't stand on ceremony. Your doctor may be naïve, but he's on your side—tell him what he needs to know.

Treatment: Simple and Effective

Assuming the diagnosis is made, what is there to do? At this point, let us all rejoice that we live in the age we do. Even 30 years ago we might have been doomed to urethral strictures and the agony of PID, depending on how the providential dice rolled. Now, once the diagnosis is made, the cure is at hand. Forget all that nonsense you have heard about clap's resistance to drugs and about killer germs invading us from abroad. There *is* some resistance on the part of the gonococcus, which we will detail, but *even after 25 years of use, penicillin is still the drug of choice.* Except for those few people with known allergies to penicillin, it can be used to effect virtually an *absolute* cure for *all* strains of gonococcus, after one strong dose.

The latest gonorrhea treatment schedules recommended by the Center for Disease Control, effective March 1972, are printed verbatim in Appendix A. These figures are not likely to change for several years, and doctors will want to study this table closely. Some things should be pointed out here to everybody.

Penicillin

The preferred drug is listed as (injectable) penicillin G, or oral ampicillin, which is a newer derivative of penicillin. The dose for men has been doubled, for penicillin, to twice the previous recommended dose. Older dosage recommendations are still found in the literature for the profession and the public; so doctors should read the doses carefully. In addition, (oral) probenecid, which is NOT an antibiotic but a regulator of certain blood and urine chemicals, should be given routinely. Probenecid has the effect of maintaining penicillin and penicillin derivatives in the body for a much longer time, instead of letting them disintegrate and be excreted in the urine. This teamwork between penicillin and probenecid was utilized when the penicillin drugs were first introduced during World War II, but was neglected when penicillan became cheap and commonplace. Doubling the dose of penicillin and adding probenecid effectively quadruples the level of penicillin in the blood in the doses previously recommended for men by the Public Health Service. The effective dose for women previously recommended by the PHS is doubled by the new recommendation for probenecid to be used with penicillin. These dosage schedules have the effect of standardizing penicillin doses for both sexes at a level well above the minimal concentration needed to kill the bacteria. *These doses absolutely and categorically cure all strains of gonococci, penicillin-resistant strains included, now known in the United States.* The problem of gonorrhea epidemics *will* be solved if everybody gets to the doctor who needs to, and if the doctor uses these strong (but not dangerous) doses. In the past, half-hearted doses and unsystematic attempts to outguess the strength of the particular gonococcus strain being treated resulted in the selective breeding and increase of resistant strains, NOT in killing all the germs. This standard dose for men and women simplifies matters for physicians and stays well ahead of drug resistance throughout the world.

Oral Ampicillin

For the first time the Public Health Service, acting through the CDC, recommends ampicillin—an oral drug—as equally effective against gonorrhea as is injectable penicillin. This makes the drug firms that manufacture ampicillin fairly hysterical with joy, and it is undoubtedly more pleasant for the patient, too. Why then, you may ask, do we not simply use the oral drugs and drop the injectable ones? The trend is definitely in that direction, but for the next few years at least, injectable penicillin has one distinct advantage: it is well known that penicillin is effective, at the dose levels given for gonorrhea, against any coincidental incubating syphilis, which may not be apparent to the physician at the time of the diagnosis of gonorrhea. In addition, ampicillin is more expensive that penicillin.

Spectinomycin and Tetracyclines

In cases of allergy to penicillin, two other drugs are recommended: spectinomycin, a new drug, and tetracycline. Of these two, from a public health point of view spectinomycin is preferable because it may be given in *one* dose under the doctor's eye. People simply cannot be relied upon to take all of several doses of medicine; once they start feeling better, they forget about the medicine, and the disease may relapse. Tetracycline requires 16 additional doses over four days. (Doxycycline, a popular tetracycline derivative, requires five doses over four days.) That's really too much to ask anyone to remember. Again, neither tetracycline nor spectinomycin is known to abort incubating syphilis; so injectable penicillin has that over them too. It should be noted that, despite rumors, fads, and pharmaceutical ballyhoo to the contrary, the rare kinds of tetracycline, such as doxycycline (e.g., Vibramycin®), do NOT have any advantage over the good old brand of plain tetracycline—except, that is, for the drug firms: doxycycline costs 25 times as much as regular tetracycline.

The complications of gonorrhea require large intravenous doses of crystalline penicillin and intensive treatment in the hospital. If you follow the simpler steps, you won't get any complications.

That's Fine, But . . .

Getting physicians to prescribe the adequate dose is not a simple thing. A study in Oregon not published as yet shows that half of the private physicians in America gave inadequate therapy even before the increase in dosage recommendations! That is why *you are better off going to public health clinics or VD clinics where they know their business.* Hopefully physician education measures will have taken effect soon, especially with the influx of $16 million into state VD programs in 1972, an election year. If your doctor doesn't give you one of the things listed in Appendix A, show it to him and ask him why.

If you get the adequate therapy, does that mean home free for you? Yes, IF you make certain of some things. If you have been sleeping with someone and intend to do so again, make sure that person and all the people he or she is sleeping with also get adequate therapy. Otherwise the germ will boomerang back to you. The single most important fact about syphilis and gonorrhea is that THERE IS NO IMMUNITY to these diseases —ever. You can get either right back again. It is essential that everybody treat this subject as thoroughly and objectively as possible. The patient has to cooperate with the doctor—go see him, take the medicine, and make sure that his contacts get to the doctor, or vice versa. The doctor *must* report infected people, *not* to the police or the law, but to a group of health workers whose job it is to contact everybody in the community with a variety of infectious diseases, not just venereal ones, to see that they are quickly eradicated. These public health workers do not gossip, and they do not confer with the police or the district attorney. All the links in the cycle of infection must be treated and cured; otherwise, the same people will be getting the same germs all over again. Fortunately, thanks to the efforts of the CDC and its doctors, like Dr. James B. Lucas, the asinine prohibitive state laws formerly denying antibiotics to minors with gonorrhea without official or parental consent are being thrown out. In over 40 states, minors are now legally able to obtain antibiotics for venereal diseases without parental consent. In those states where such absurd laws still exist, in an apparent attempt to deny the problem by preventing its cure, doctors should give the appropriate therapy to their patients for all diseases at all ages. Hopefully, soon all of our states will wake up; most of the laws in the 40 states were enacted in the last two years.

Assuming, then, that you and the people you sleep

with are all treated at the same time, you are "safe" within 24 hours of complete treatment to go out and enjoy yourself without fear of infecting anyone. Nevertheless, you should go back for a follow-up culture the next week just to be sure you are not in that less-than-1-percent group requiring additional therapy.

Prevention

Condoms

An old Indian saying goes: "White man fool Indian once, shame on white man. White man fool Indian twice, shame on Indian." Consider yourself warned. The best way to deal with the clap is to prevent it. This involves knowing all the symptoms in yourself and your sexual partners. Unfortunately, there is no foolproof method at this time to prevent getting gonorrhea. Well over 90 percent of the time, the condom or "rubber" does prevent transmission of the gonococcus in all kinds of sex. But use of the condom has dropped with overreliance on The Pill to prevent babies, antibiotics to fall back on, and the desire of most people these days to do it "natural." Using condoms is a good way to prevent the spread of many venereal diseases; so use them if they don't bother you.

Some simple procedures help avoid gonorrhea. Don't have sex with a full bladder. This tends to hurt the organs mechanically and thus make them less resistant to germs. (Remember, just because you contract a goncoccus doesn't mean it will be able to survive and grow on you.) And since the germs may travel up the urethras of both sexes, urinating after sex helps somewhat to flush them out. The urine is sterile in normal people, and by urinating you irrigate yourself beautifully. The primeval male who rolls over and goes to sleep after he "does it" is at a disadvantage here. Taking a good soapy shower or using a bidet helps remove any germs. Douching is ineffective and should not become routine, for reasons that are explained in Chapter Eight.

DON'T Take Antibiotics "Just in Case"

One way to prevent gonorrhea is to take *adequate* doses of antibiotics before or just after sex. But few people know how much is enough! You should NOT do it unless you are a competent physician. First, antibiotics are obtained only with a prescription, so that the antibiotics available to most people are old ones growing useless on the shelf. Additionally, chronic self-administration of tetracyclines or penicillin can cause drug resistance, allergies, and even liver disease. It is widely held that the major cause of increasing resistance to drugs by gonococci over the past 20 years has been sloppy and amateur doses of antibiotics. Properly administered large doses such as those recommended by the United States Public Health Service Venereal Disease Branch and given in Appendix A kill off virtually all the germs, even of resistant strains. Inadequate doses tend to kill off the weak strains and let the resistant strains take the field. It is very bad medicine for people to go around popping pills like Ju-Jubes. Relying on pills to cure any ailment establishes a lazy and dangerous attitude that may result in further physical illness. Inadequate doses may quiet the disease temporarily, but the problem may rear up later, uglier and more complicated than before. For example, self-administered erratic doses of drugs for gonorrhea might prevent a local vaginitis in a woman, only to let the gonococci spread quietly and lead to PID, peritonitis, sterility, and hysterectomy later. Altogether, the best thing to do is to keep yourself alert for symptoms without playing Dr. Kildare.

Prevention on a Massive Scale

If everybody did all of this, would the venereal disease epidemic end? Absolutely not. The reason is that all those asymptomatic, untroubled, and indifferent men and women would still be running around like so many sexual Typhoid Marys, spreading the clap without knowing it. What is needed is routine screening of *every patient who sees a doctor* on routine checkups or for any other symptom. Everyone from the age of sexual maturity to 60 should have certain routine tests performed regularly, even if he has sex only once a month, like Tristram Shandy's father. All women undergoing routine gynecology exams for Pap smears should have vaginal cultures and rectal cultures for gonorrhea done just as routinely. It is so easy to obtain these crucial cultures during a routine pelvic exam. And it is so essential. Estimates on the number of infected women are staggering. Of the 2,200,000 estimated cases last year, 700,000 were women. Since 9 out of 10 women stay asymptomatic, there are possibly millions of women walking around with no symptoms but with active gonorrhea, progressing inexorably to PID. These women can have all the serious complications and can infect millions of men, who in turn infect other women (and men), and so on. The only way doctors will ever find them is to do routine gonococci cultures on *every woman who comes into the office for any reason.* Sexually active women should insist on gonorrhea cultures routinely with each pelvic exam and Pap smear, that is, at least once a year.

Similar checks should be done yearly on all homosexual men in the throat and rectum. It is a good idea for doctors to do a rectal culture for gonococci at each rectal exam, no matter what the person's sexual preference seems to be. Certainly whenever the person goes to the doctor complaining of the possibility of gonorrhea, the rectum should be cultured for gonococci if they are not found in the penis. As the patient, you should urge your doctor to do these things if he or she doesn't automatically do them.

Private physicians must begin to report gonorrhea to the public health caseworkers, local, state, and United States public health personnel, who still must do the shoe leather work to aid exposed and infected people.

The "Vaccine," the "Blood Test," and Other Rainbows

There is much talk about a "blood test" to diagnose the clap or a "vaccine" to prevent it, but neither is anywhere near realization at the present. There is in fact no reliable blood test for gonococci. To have a blood test for any particular germ, that germ must have certain kinds of carbohydrate and protein that stimulate the body to form antibodies that provide immunity. These germ particles are called antigens; and with the body's reactive antibodies, they are detectable by laboratory "blood tests." Whereas the syphilis germ stimulates a large antibody reaction, and variations of the syphilis blood test (the Wassermann) have existed for over 50 years, nothing strong enough to prompt dependable antibody detection has been evolved for the gonococcus. Recently Drs. Tom Buchanan and Emil

Gottschlik of Rockefeller University in New York City have discovered that of the four cultural types of gonococci known, the two disease-producing types alone have hairlike particles that are found only during infection. These projections cause the reactive production of antibodies in the human serum, unlike any fragment of the gonococcus previously known. These gentlemen are presently working on a blood test based on these findings, which have excited even the most skeptical infectious disease experts. A clinical test is just now underway. If it succeeds, there may at last be a blood test for gonorrhea, which, if routinely administered, could identify every single case of gonococcal infection. This would be a major breakthrough in diagnosis for public health.

The same problem of a lack of consistent antibody-provoking substances in the gonococcus has obstructed the development of a gonorrhea vaccine, which would certainly be one of the great clinical events of the century and would merit a round trip to Stockholm, courtesy of the Nobel committee. The basis for successful vaccines, like Salk's and Sabin's for poliomyelitis, has been to alter disease-producing germs in such a way that they cause production of antibodies in the host, and thus immunity, but not the destructive changes that cause disease. The polio virus causes nervous system destruction and also triggers production of antibodies that fight off the virus—but only after the damage has been done. Salk and Sabin separately treated strains of polio viruses that caused no damage but had the antigenic requirements to stimulate immunity. But in gonorrhea, there is no immunity! Even after you get the disease, you never become immune. Nevertheless, there have been attempts to take gonococcal fragments and add immunity-boosting agents to try to develop immunity. Dr. Louis Greenberg of Canada is one of those working on a field trial of just such a boosted "vaccine" in the Northwest Territories.

We wish all these doctors well who are working in this most humane field of research. The doctor who frees sexual activity from the stigmas of fear and disease that have crippled it these many centuries will have gone a long way toward civilizing mankind at last.

Gonorrhea of the Newborn

Two twists in the complex of gonorrhea syndromes have been saved until now in order not to distract from the logical progression that the story of gonorrhea, for the most part, follows. The first is *ophthalmia neonatorum,* or gonococcal infection arising during birth in babies' eyes. As the infant slides through the vagina of a woman infected with gonorrhea, the bacteria can get into the eyes and cause a reddening of the eyes (*conjunctivitis*) that can spread throughout the structure of the eyeball and cause total destruction of the cornea and blindness within 24 hours. Hospitals have used silver nitrate solution at birth routinely to prevent this condition, but the number of cases has somehow been increasing in recent years because of the increase in gonorrhea cases. Treatment involves isolation of the infected newborn (to prevent nursery epidemics) and injections of penicillin. Because of this tragic disease entity it is recommended that all pregnant women be cultured for gonococci by their obstetrician during the first and last months of pregnancy.

Nongonococcal Urethritis (Nonspecific Urethritis)

A large number of men who are sexually active suffer from a chronic condition variously known by the two above names. This condition is receiving a great deal of attention these days because of the number of patients who seem to have it, and because there is a great deal of controversy in medical circles as to exactly what nonspecific urethritis is. The typical complaint is that after almost every sexual encounter, the man has burning, itching, and general discomfort in the penis. There may be some thin drainage, or even a pus discharge. The disturbance may be less dramatic than that of gonorrhea, with less drainage and less burning on urination, but it tends to persist without diminishing. Of course the first thing that comes to mind the first time it happens is gonorrhea, and doctors must culture the discharge for gonococcal germs. However, in cases that come to be labeled nonspecific urethritis, no gonococcus is ever cultured. In fact, the diagnosis is made by excluding gonorrhea and all other provable causes. In many cases of "nonspecific urethritis" special culture techniques have isolated rare germs like *Chlamydia* and *Mycoplasma,* which are halfway between bacteria and viruses. These special culture techniques are unavailable at most clinical centers. Many medical experts feel, however, that if cases of nonspecific urethritis were searched still more thoroughly, using massage of the prostate and other manipulations to coax the germs from crypts and recesses in the genitourinary tracts, gonococci would be found. One recent study shows just that.

The central fact, whatever the infectious agent, is that the *clinical* picture of nonspecific urethritis is different from that of gonorrhea. Although the pain is less, and pus is usually absent, and there are no known complications or systemic body manifestations of nongonococcal urethritis, the itching and burning may persist for months, flaring up after occasional episodes of sexual intercourse. Although one dose of penicillin quickly cures the clap, large doses of penicillin are often unable to clear up nonspecific urethritis. Tetracyclines and other antibiotics are used, and treatment simply becomes a long siege until the right drug is found and taken in sufficient quantities. This sort of diagnosis and treatment, in which the doctor cannot pinpoint the offending germ for his patient, is frustrating for both concerned. A good deal of patience is required from both. Every effort must be made to find a gonococcus on *repeated* attempts, and the patient must take all his medicines whenever directed. It may be necessary to take some antibiotics after each episode of sex to prevent new flare-ups, as the doctor directs.

The consoling points are these. First, nonspecific urethritis cannot be transferred from men to women. It seems to be a problem pertinent only to the male anatomy and is at least in some instances due to recurring mechanical irritation stirring up some infection hidden in the recesses of the male urethra, or possibly the prostate or seminal vesicles. If a "nonspecific urethritis" is caught by the female partner of a man supposedly suffering from this disorder, gonococci can often be cultured from the woman, and the diagnosis and therapy are promptly changed. Second, there are no known complications of nonspecific urethritis, and the problem remains localized to the penis as a limited irritation. Third, eventually, with treatment over a period of weeks or months, the infections *are* cured. Cure is quickened if some effort is made to use lubricants during sex and to avoid reddening or other mechanical irritation of the penis during intercourse.

Chapter Five:
SYPHILIS

Introduction

During the great epidemic of a certain disease that swept Europe in the early sixteenth century, a poet invented a shepherd who came down with the affliction and named him "Syphilis" because it had a nice ring to it. The name stuck. Since then, a great deal of attention has been given to syphilis by word of mouth and in print. Much of what is on record about syphilis has been silly at best; at worst, it has greatly harmed the cause of health. Every wit, every moralist, every politician with some bone to pick has bent the subject to his own purpose. Chauvinists have exploited it: the English referred to it condescendingly as the French disease, the French shrugged it off as the Italian disease, and the Italians gestured at whoever was then invading their country. Overzealous preachers have pointed at syphilis as a curse of God and a "punishment" for sex. European historians have looked down on the "Indians" of the Caribbean for giving syphilis to Columbus and starting the epidemic in Europe, and apologists for the Indians say Columbus gave it to them. Now medical authorities, in a gush of racial peacemaking, say that syphilis is an ancient disease that every society has had and point to the Old Testament as "proof."

What difference does it make who gave it to whom, historically, nationally, or personally, even today? The fog of history will never part to let us see the truth of thousands of years ago; so why should we waste our time speculating over the angels on this pinhead? What we do care about is the way it affects us today: the way the disease has evolved, and the methods we have developed to treat it. It is time that people stopped scoring political points about syphilis and started getting rid of it altogether.

A hundred years ago, Sir William Osler intoned, "Who knows syphilis, knows medicine," because the disease was so prevalent and mimicked so many other diseases. Not so today. Dr. Zoltan Ovary, internationally renowned professor of immunology from New York University, who has seen a lot of medicine during his career, told me emphatically, "Syphilis has changed so much! People used to drop dead in the streets from syphilis. It is totally different now." Syphilis used to run through and destroy a person in a few weeks, after producing rashes, fevers, and pus-filled infections all over the body. Complications came soon after the primary chancres (first-stage sores), and lives were shortened by 20 to 30 years, *if* the original attack was survived.

Why does a disease change from the severe continent-wide epidemic of the sixteenth century to the manageable disease it is now? There are several reasons we can understand. First, there is a natural give-and-take of host-parasite relationships that has killed off the more destructive strains of the syphilis organism, the *Treponema pallidum.* In order to survive as a species over the long run, bacteria and viruses have to keep their victims alive long enough to reproduce inside them and get picked up by another human victim. In this way the cycle keeps going. The stronger, killer germs simply killed off their victims too quickly and were not kept going from person to person. Therefore, these fatal strains have disappeared from the picture, with a grudging bow to Darwin and natural selection.

In addition, medical treatment may have altered the syphilis strains. In the early 1900s heavy metals—arsenic, bismuth, and mercury—were used as therapy, and they weakened some of the stronger strains. Lately penicillin has radically altered the syphilis population, killing off many of the more devastating subtypes of syphilis and changing the clinical picture of the disease markedly. Today, *even untreated,* the course of syphilis is much more benign than it used to be. In one-third of untreated syphilis victims no complications are ever noticed. When complications do arise, there is a delay period of at least 10 years during which nothing seems wrong. Nevertheless, there are still awful consequences to risk with this disease.

Misconceptions

A complete list of folk legends about syphilis would make up a horror show that would put Edgar Allan Poe to shame. We can't go into them all, but some misconceptions are too popular to go uncorrected. First, the terms *syphilis* and *venereal disease* are NOT the same; syphilis is of course only one of many diseases contracted largely through venery, or lovemaking.

Syphilis is a specific set of disease problems caused by one sovereign set of bacteria that has nothing to do with any other set of germs. You can get syphilis umpteen times and never get gonorrhea, and vice versa. There is no connection between the two except that they prefer the same environment.

Then there's the false notion that, once you get syphilis, you're marked for life, like Hester Prynne with that "A." Nonsense. Your body can be pure as a virgin's one day after adequate treatment. Furthermore, you NEVER become immune to syphilis; you can get it again and again. You must keep constantly alert so that if you ever get it, and *each time* you get it, you take the right treatment and do not slide into that dangerous "grace" period before latent disaster sets in. And let's have no recriminations or pointing fingers at whoever "gave" it to you. These are as useless as pointing the finger at Columbus or his Indian friends. We are all in this together. Make sure your lovers are reached by public health personnel who can *help* them, cure their disease, and prevent the disease from getting back to you. This is a health problem and must be treated as such, thoroughly and dispassionately. There is no "blame" to getting sick.

People who have had syphilis can marry and have lovely, normal children and lead lovely, normal lives if they receive simple antibiotic therapy. You do not have to abstain from sex for any more than a day or two after you are treated for syphilis; check this with your doctor.

Contrary to what you heard in the cloakroom of Mrs. Whoozit's fourth-grade class at recess, your thing will NOT fall off, no matter which thing it is. This pernicious folktale has been causing nightmares for impressionable kids for centuries and probably could be traced back to the ancient confusion of syphilis with leprosy. Perhaps our generation can bury it.

You do NOT automatically go blind or crazy from syphilis. Yes, there are severe nervous system and ophthalmic complications resulting from syphilis, but in no case would these occur without 20 years or so of your ignoring your health and having exceptionally bad luck besides. If you ever get adequate treatment for syphilis *at any time after you get it,* you will always prevent these and all other complications that have not already occurred. Nevertheless, even in untreated persons, the risk of mental deterioration or blindness in old age as a complication of untreated syphilis is small. Nevertheless, costs being what they are, the Public Health Service has estimated that the taxpayer shells out $46 million a year to keep some people in mental hospitals who developed mental and nervous system aberrations many years after primary syphilis.

If you are already aware of these facts, good. Unfortunately many people are not. Please remember that syphilis is a disease like any other bacterial disease, with a wide variety of possible effects on you. The damage done depends on many interrelating factors. You don't automatically get sick just because you come across or acquire a germ. Your own natural strength and reserve, your natural and acquired immunities, your state of nutrition, your daily physical and emotional stress balance with the strength of the particular germs you're fighting, the number of germs you've acquired, the coincidental use of antibiotics or drugs for other reasons, and so on. You are probably harboring thousands of bacteria in your throat that would kill many other people with the right weaknesses, but you have learned to live with them peacefully for years.

It is the same with syphilis. There is no neat, inevitable package of doom awaiting you if you come into contact with someone with syphilis. The germs may not get to you. If they do land physically in or on your body, you may fight them off and get no infection. Or if they do take hold, they may never do any noticeable damage and then get killed off with no harmful aftereffects. Most commonly, if you are infected (that is, if the germs *do* gain a foothold in your own private ecosystem), you will get a primary chancre; but you still may not get any complications later in life. The thing to remember is that syphilis is now easy to understand and to treat. If you pay attention to this chapter and apply it to yourself, you can avoid *all* severe problems associated with syphilis.

Sources and Risks

The whole disease pattern of syphilis has changed radically over the last 400 years, and especially in the last 30. As a result, informed opinion about the statistics of the disease varies, even in adjacent offices of infectious disease experts. Twenty-five thousand new cases of all kind of infectious syphilis were reported by state and local health agencies and private doctors to the U.S. Public Health Service last year, and many more new cases will develop but remain untreated each year. The number of treated cases that go unreported by physicians to health services is estimated at around 100,000 people. That means that there are (1) 10 to 20 times as many cases of gonorrhea as of syphilis, (2) a great many people running around with untreated syphilis, and (3) a great many people treated for syphilis whose infected contacts have never been treated.

There seems to be little connection between the risk of getting gonorrhea and the risk of getting syphilis. Only 3 percent of people coming to the doctor for gonorrhea have syphilis. Statistics indicate that certain urban areas have extremely high rates of syphilis and low rates of gonorrhea (New York City; San Juan; and Dayton, Ohio); some have high gonorrhea rates and low rates of syphilis (New Haven, Charlotte, and Memphis); some, indeed most, have high rates of both (Atlanta, Washington, San Francisco, Newark, Baltimore, and Hartford); and some have low rates of both (Honolulu, San Diego, Phoenix, San Antonio, Tulsa, Albuquerque, and Pittsburgh). In general, urban areas and more populated states have higher rates of both than the vast open prairie and mountain states. This is easily understandable. But rates are up all over the country, and since people move around a lot these days, the problem is truly a national one.

The incidence of both syphilis and gonorrhea among blacks is *reported* to be much higher than among whites. But "reported" is a loaded word: Blacks are poorer than whites and go to public health facilities rather than to more costly private physicians. Public doctors have a much higher rate of reporting cases to the USPHS than do private doctors. Because of this bias of the figures, some doctors—indeed some experts—still think that gonorrhea is a "higher-class" disease than syphilis. This is simply not true. What is true is that the more people you have sex with, the more likely you are to get either disease or both. Very promiscuous groups of people, such as male and female prostitutes and some male homosexuals, have a much higher rate of infection for both diseases. It is estimated that in some areas as many as 40 to 50 percent of new syphilis cases occur in male homosexuals. The notion that blacks get VD more often than whites because they are more promiscuous is sheer racist stereotype.

Statistics are interesting to you, of course, only as they apply to you. If you have sex with a syphilitic person and acquire the disease, your chances are these:

One-third of the time, nothing will happen. One-third of the time you will develop a persistently reactive blood test, but the disease will stop there. One-third of the time you will go on, if untreated, to severe complications late in life such as an aortic aneurysm or heart trouble, brain or spinal cord damage. These poor odds and the descriptions below will hopefully lead you to conclude something we suggest much farther on in this chapter.

Symptoms and Signs of Syphilis

Introduction

Syphilis is far more insidious than gonorrhea. With gonorrhea, symptoms are so severe in most men that they seek medical attention immediately. In women the clap more often than not goes unnoticed. This means that most men are treated, while women languish with gonorrhea unknowing and untreated, serving as the major reservoir for the spread of gonorrhea. In syphilis the wounds or "lesions" are most often PAINLESS in BOTH sexes, so that the tendency is to ignore the first signs of the disease until, 20 years later, you get clobbered. The chancre (SHANG-ker), the wart, the rash of syphilis can hide unseen in crevices of the body. If you spot one of these, you may think it so small, so painless, so unimportant looking that you ignore it. These little signs go away after a while, but the germs linger within you, causing great structural damage in the unfortunate third of victims in whom the disease continues unabated by any natural defense or chance. Thus with syphilis you are much more likely NOT to notice the problem than with gonorrhea whether you are a man or a woman, and you are much more likely to go on to severe problems with syphilis.

Part One: Primary Syphilis (First-Stage Syphilis)

The first stage of syphilis involves skin changes or lesions at the site of sexual contact with the germ. First changes are noticed after an incubation period of 10 to 90 days, usually averaging about three weeks after acquiring the germs. (Incidentally, since the incubation period for gonorrhea is much shorter, you may have seen a doctor and been treated for gonorrhea long before you develop signs of syphilis obtained from the same sexual partner. Treatment for gonorrhea aborts the incubating syphilis bacteria, but you must return in a few weeks to make sure that your blood test for syphilis stays negative.) You may pass through the primary stage of syphilis and NOT notice a chancre at all, especially if you are a woman and the primary lesion is internal.

The syphilis spirochetes corkscrew into the skin where sexual contact was the most vigorous. Even the usual friction of sexual intercourse affords the syphilis germs easy entrance to the body. If you rely on smooth, unscratched skin to protect you, you will be greatly disappointed. As the organisms enter the skin, the area involved becomes swollen and inflamed as the body tries unsuccessfully to defend itself.

The primary sore—the chancre—begins as a dull-red flat spot, usually less than a dime in diameter, and then becomes elevated and blistery-looking. The surface soon erodes and takes on a smooth, round, clearly defined ulcerous appearance. The ulcer usually does not bleed, does not drain pus, and looks generally clean and harmless. It does not smell, and *it does not hurt.* There may be one ulcer or several. The most common sites are the penis near its head, or on the shaft; the outside vulva (*labia majora*); and the inside vulva (*labia minora*). The lips, the tongue, the skin outside the rectum, inside the anus, inside the cheeks, and even the tonsils are also vulnerable. Chancres inside the vagina are rare; at the far end of the vaginal vault, they are common. The chancre may ooze a little clear fluid or become secondarily infected, but in general it is so painless that it does not alarm you unless you know what it is. Chancres that occur on nongenital parts of the body, such as the finger or the tongue, may be noticed but not thought of in connection with any sexual activity and thus may be passed off as fever blisters or even pimples.

The syphilitic chancre heals very slowly over three to eight weeks. It leaves a thin, colorless scar that may be so inconspicuous that neither you nor your doctor ever notices it. One clue to its origin is that it is quite firm and hard when you touch it, like a smooth scar in formation. This tough, painless quality distinguishes it from the painful "soft chancre" of chancroid disease, which is another infectious disease discussed in another chapter.

In most cases, these few symptoms are the only clues you have to primary syphilis. You can pass through it and not know it, like Delaware. There is no pain, even during sex, or when you urinate. You do not lose your desire or ability to have sex, and *there is never any connection between sexual impotence and syphilis.* If you do notice a blister or a sore of any kind on your private parts, go to a doctor at once. He will be able to tell you whether it is due to syphilis, or chancroid, or herpes virus of the genitals, or whatever it is—or isn't. He will squeeze a few drops of fluid from the lesion, to find out if it is syphilitic and will examine those drops under a dark-field microscope to make the diagnosis. Your blood test will usually NOT have turned positive in this short period of time, if you go to the doctor within a few weeks of developing the chancre. If the dark-field exam is negative at first, the doctor will repeat the test, but all too frequently he may assume you have the disease and treat you for it, to assure your safety.

In all primary cases, if you have gotten a strong dose of syphilis, the germs may already have spread to lymph glands in your groin, on one or both sides. In most people, this painful lymph node swelling may not be noticeable even if it does occur.

Part Two: Secondary Syphilis (Second-Stage Syphilis)

If you are treated for primary syphilis, the whole matter will stop right there. Otherwise the infection will progress and show up later in the secondary stage and/or as tertiary syphilis. Secondary symptoms follow primary ones—if at all—three to eight weeks later. In many cases the chancre will have been long gone, making it difficult to connect the second-stage symptoms with syphilis. Secondary syphilis is not a local reaction, as is the chancre, but results from generalized spread of the germs through the blood to many other organs. This wide spread accounts for the variability of symptoms.

The Rash. The most frequent secondary symptom is the "rash" of syphilis. Unfortunately there is no single type of rash we can describe. Secondary syphilis can mimic any other kind of rash. It may comprise a few barely noticeable "pimples" or "heat rash" eruptions around the genital area or the site of the primary chancre itself. It may be limited to one or two places on the body with no particular distribution. If may consist of numerous delicate pale pink, pinhead-sized bumps that lie flat on the skin, like measles. Such low-lying bumps turn colorless when you press down on them and are found chiefly on the upper body.

Much more commonly, the rash may have larger bumps the size of peas that rise above the skin level and turn darker red, involving wide areas of the body. These blisters are round, well marginated, and symmetrically distributed over the trunk, arms, legs, palms, soles, and face. They feel hard when pressed. The individual blisters vary in size and elevation.

These raised areas involve a hyperreaction of the skin to the germs seeded within it and can become large and fleshy in moist areas, especially around the scrotum or vulva, on the thighs, and around the anus. In these crotch areas they become large and fleshy and are called syphilitic warts. These moist "warts" ooze serum and are the most infectious lesions of syphilis, after the chancre. The technical term for them is *condylomata lata,* or flat warts. They must be distinguished from nonsyphilitic "venereal warts" that are found on many people. (Nonsyphilitic warts are called *condylomata acuminata,* for the record.) Syphilitic warts are redder or darker than the syphilis skin changes found elsewhere on the body. With serum oozing out they can become superficially infected by other bacteria and drain pus and are smelly and objectionable.

Syphilitic blisters can occur on the head, where they cause patchy shedding of hair. On the palms and soles of the feet they take on the tough nature of the skin already there and resemble dark calluses. They DO itch. As they dry up, scabs can form on them, and the whole picture can feign psoriasis. In particularly undernourished or weak patients these blisters may become extensive.

Dreadful as they sound, these skin eruptions heal by themselves, leaving very small discolored spots, if anything. Today severe skin manifestations of syphilis are rare; a few hundred years ago, syphilitic "pox" was feared as we fear smallpox. To us, the chief trouble with secondary syphilis is that the moist lesions are highly infectious for anyone who touches them.

Systemic Symptoms (Symptoms Throughout the Body). In the secondary phase the victim can have symptoms affecting his whole body. These symptoms are usually not severe. The most common is the rash, but others are also frequent. Headache, general blah feeling, lack of appetite, and weight loss may occur. A slight fever may come and go, along with sore throat or hoarseness. Swelling in the lymph nodes may spread from the groin to other nodes in the armpits, neck, or trunk. In general, these symptoms are not severe and may be ignored or attributed to "the flu" or some "virus that's going around."

A visible secondary symptom is the "mucous patch," a painless ulcer on the delicate membranes inside the mouth, cheek, tongue, or vagina, or around the penis. These grayish white patches may form ulcers about the size of dimes; like chancres they usually do not hurt, but they get where they are not by direct touching but by spread through the blood from another source. If patches develop on the vocal cords, you get hoarse.

Syphilis organisms can spread directly to the liver and cause jaundice and hepatitis (inflammation of the liver) in the secondary or even the late primary period. This whole subject is poorly explored, and there are so few proven cases in the literature that expert opinion on this matter simply does not exist, but the alert doctor should keep this possibility in mind when an unusual hepatitis occurs.

Diagnosis. Thus the doctor faced with a rash that looks like measles, German measles, drug reactions, seborrhea, typhoid fever, pityriasis rosea, smallpox, chickenpox, leprosy, tuberculosis, hives, psoriasis, acne, ecthyma, pyoderma, fungus infections, impetigo, lichen planus, granuloma annulare, ringworm, simple baldness, or simple venereal warts may actually be confronting the secondary rash of syphilis! No wonder Sir William Osler was so impressed.

But do not despair. Your part in this drama is very simple. If you get an unusual rash—whether you are sexually active or not—go to a doctor and show it to him. If pressed, you may recall having had something that fits the description of a primary chancre some time ago. Most doctors in America faced with a new rash of any kind will test you with a blood test for syphilis, usually the "VDRL" test which is the Venereal Diseases Research Laboratory version of the "Wassermann" now used. The doctor will be able to make an absolute diagnosis. By the time secondary syphilis occurs, the body has developed a reaction to the syphilis organisms sufficient to cause a positive blood test. So no matter what form your secondary rash takes, if you get to a skilled doctor you will get the correct diagnosis. You should volunteer your sexual history to put him on the right track. All forms of secondary syphilis respond to the same single dose of penicillin in nearly every case. In a few cases, a second dose will be needed. Within 24 hours of the injection, any skin infection will have died off, and you will be noninfectious to those around you. (Please see the section on treatment below.) So, despite the repulsive descriptions of secondary syphilis, this part of the story is guaranteed to have a happy ending if you get proper medical attention. Warning: oral or regular penicillin is NOT recommended for syphilis at this stage; so don't play doctor for yourself or your friends.

Part Three: Tertiary Syphilis (Third-Stage or Late Syphilis)

Introduction. If a person leaves the secondary stage of syphilis untreated, he passes into a never-never land and risks a dreadful outcome. After a long latent period, tertiary syphilis can rob a man of his strength, his upright stature, his muscle control, his mind, and, often gruesomely, his life. In one-third of all people with untreated syphilis, one or more of these fates is almost certain, even in an era when syphilis is not as bad as it used to be. Of course, one can always hope to be among those who manage to get home free. It is not worth the risk, considering the little effort required to be safe and sure.

After the symptoms of second-stage syphilis disappear, nothing noticeable happens for years. The disease is still very much alive, but it shows itself ONLY if you hunt it out with blood tests. Infection may thus be detected because the patient has to get a blood test before marrying, or before giving blood, or for some fortunate bureaucratic routine. In suspected cases during this latent period, the spinal fluid should be examined as well as the blood. Although spinal taps are simple and not dangerous, they are certainly more trouble than looking for the disease at an earlier period. People are not infectious to anyone else in the latent stage, except for pregnant women, who even though showing no signs of the disease can pass it on in a lethal dose to their fetuses. As soon as the late symptoms start showing up, you have by definition left the "latent" period and entered the tertiary stage.

If at any time an infected person in the latent stage is treated, his infection can still be totally cured, although the blood tests often do not revert completely to normal. That means all the syphilis germs can be killed and all future damage totally avoided. However, since syphilis bacteria begin to inflict gross anatomical damage during this period, any damage already done by the time treatment is effected cannot be reversed. Obviously, the earlier you get to a doctor, the better off you are. And the sooner doctors do routine blood tests on *all* their patients, with or without complaints, the earlier these time bomb cases can be detected and defused.

The Gumma. It is not within the province of this book to describe all the lesions of tertiary syphilis. Osler's injunction reminds us that nearly every severe disease of man can be imitated very well by the devious and patient syphilis germ. Thirty years ago hundreds of medical volumes were written exclusively about tertiary syphilis, and although the number of cases has decreased markedly, examples of each type of syphilis can still be found. It would be presumptuous for this our modest sampler to try to scan the chessboard of moves syphilis can inflict on the unsuspecting tertiary patient.

However, if you understand the basic destructive pattern of the long-acting syphilis germs, you can well imagine the kinds of damage done. The characteristic late lesion of the syphilis bacteria is known as the *gumma.* A gumma is an area of normal tissue that has been destroyed, replaced by narrow scar tissue, and compressed by surrounding normal tissue. Gummas may replace large chunks of the liver, causing jaundice, cirrhosis, and death. They can erode large skin surfaces and look like diabetic ulcers or large bedsores. Bumps and nodules and areas of discoloration can occur on the skin. Parts of the tongue can become scarred. Bones can be eroded and gross disfigurement of the extremities can occur.

Syphilis spirochetes can cause obliteration of tiny blood vessels in the brain and cause psychosis and senility. A President of the United States, not of recent times, died of this complication.

Indeed, there is not a cubic inch of the body that the syphilis germs, given 20 or 30 years with a free hand, cannot reach and destroy. Even today, 2,000 people a year—or one out of five untreated patients—die of late complications of syphilis. Two hundred and fifty neurosyphilitic psychotics are admitted each year to VA hospitals across the country. This is a tragic legacy in an enlightened country where antibiotics are easy to get, and we should do better.

Cardiovascular Syphilis (Heart and Blood Vessel Syphilis). More than 1 out of 10 people with late, untreated syphilis dies of complications to the heart and arteries from syphilis. In most cases, neither the patient nor his doctor ever knows why. It is hard to imagine that that angelic, white-haired grandmother was once a lusty young wench; and autopsies are often omitted or inconclusive. Cardiovascular syphilis is commoner in blacks than in whites, and in men than in women. Most people who get it develop clinical signs within 20 years. In about a fourth of the people with cardiovascular syphilis, nervous system changes also occur. Diagnosing the condition during life demands careful clinical examination with special radiographic studies in addition to serological tests.

The heart symptoms of syphilis are like those of all

other heart disease, including shortness of breath, chest pains, palpitations, irregular heartbeats, poor exercise tolerance, and so on. Gummas of the heart destroy the muscles and valves, diminishing the effectiveness of the heart as a pump and setting up patterns of heart failure like those of rheumatic heart disease.

Syphilis germs over the years invade the lining of the wall of the aorta—the main blood vessel—in the chest where it leaves the heart and bends downward. The aorta balloons out into thin-walled malformations called aneurysms that eventually burst. There are most often NO warning signs in this condition, although occasionally the sac becomes so large that it presses on other structures within the chest and causes chest pain.

When syphilitic changes of the aorta are detected, present technology sometimes permits replacement of the defective part with synthetic arteries. In the hands of expert cardiovascular surgeons, this procedure has become almost commonplace. Changes to the heart muscle cannot be repaired, but unyielding or incompetent valves in the heart can be replaced by synthetic devices with a fairly good outcome.

Neurosyphilis. Syphilis germs allowed to remain in the body untreated attack the blood vessels, the supporting structures, and the very substance of the central nervous system itself.

Brain. Syphilis of the brain can focus on the lining of the brain (the meninges), the blood vessels, or the brain cells. In *secondary* syphilis, bacteria can inflame the lining of the brain causing acute *meningitis* that very quickly threatens the life of the patient. Symptoms are those of any other kind of meningitis: headache, nausea, and vomiting, convulsions, paralysis, and mental confusion. In *tertiary* syphilis, meningitis can develop as a *chronic* disorder, with the same symptoms appearing gradually.

Syphilis in the blood vessels of the brain can block essential arteries and result in strokes that lead to paralysis, sensation loss, mental deterioration, and even death.

When the brain tissue is attacked directly, the results are pathetic. The clinical syndrome is known as GPI—general paralysis of the insane—although this cruelly accurate name is fading from favor. Symptoms progress from slight and vague eccentricities to total mental incompetence. At first, the patient may become irritable and lose his concentration, interest, and memory. He may develop antisocial or even criminal behavior. Headaches may occur, and all reasoning ability is lost. Convulsions, mild paralysis, and slurred speech develop. Usually the person is unaware of what is happening to him, and it is his horrified family who bring him to the attention of a physican. There is little satisfaction in knowing that Uncle So-and-So is crazy because of syphilis and not just "plain crazy."

Spinal Cord. In the spinal cord, most destruction is made on the nervous tissue directly. Destruction of nerve cells leads to a condition called *tabes dorsalis* (TA-beeze dor-SA-lis). Classic examples of this disorder may be seen in any mental hospital in the country, and the picture is not a pretty one. Symptoms rarely appear earlier than 10 to 20 years after the first infection; even then, they develop gradually. They include characteristic "lightning pains" that stab through the legs and, less typically, through the back and arms. As time goes on, they become extremely severe. Funny feelings and cramps accompany the lightning pains in the legs. The victim loses all ability to balance his body with his eyes closed and has a peculiar gait. (This is one of the easiest gaits medical students learn to imitate.) Bladder and bowel and sexual impairments arise from destruction of the lower spinal roots. One out of five patients with tabes dorsalis becomes gradually blind. Impairment of facial functions also is common.

Although changes like these cannot be reversed, the unfortunate person who has them can still profit from therapy with penicillin to arrest the progression of the disease and prevent total disaster, although blindness may progress despite therapy at this stage.

Tabes dorsalis can occur along with GPI or other late syphilitic problems. Both must be distinguished from vitamin deficiencies, alcoholism (which is often coexistent), lead poisoning, diabetes, poliomyelitis, spinal cord tumors, multiple sclerosis, and so on.

Congenital Syphilis

As dreadful as these late complications of syphilis are, they are not the worst results of syphilis. St. Augustine distinguished between *vice,* which is doing something bad to yourself, and *crime,* which is doing something bad to someone else. With present-day information and technology, surely it is a crime, in ethical if not legal terms, to pass on the destructive germs of syphilis to one's unborn child. Yet this is unwittingly done. Last year there were 400 children born in this country with syphilis passed on to them by their infected mothers, most of whom did not have symptoms and had not bothered to get a blood test. Many of these children have severe physical disfigurements, as well as mental retardation, blindness, and deafness. There is a certain beggar on Fifth Avenue, with a crushed and twisted nose and the glazed gray, unseeing eyes of the totally blind, who is a classic example of this almost unbearably tragic disease. Obviously her mother could not have known what was going on inside her; it would be nice to think that we can educate everyone to obtain regular syphilis blood tests and thus avoid being the unwilling instrument of such hardship.

The syphilis bacteria can devastate the growing fetus, as its cell mass doubles and triples every hour. Indeed in 30 percent of infected fetuses, a spontaneous miscarriage occurs and life is ended altogether. In another large percentage, the deformed fetus is stillborn. In those who survive, there is no organ that cannot be altered at birth; grossly deformed bones and soft tissue structure may ensue, with characteristic defects running down the midline of the body, on the nose, the palate, and the chest. Long bones often develop a "saber" appearance.

Massive doses of penicillin to the noticeably infected infant at birth are often not enough to save the life of the child. Even if the child's life is saved, any damage already done cannot be reversed; but further damage can be prevented.

In addition, a normal-appearing child can develop gross alterations of anatomy and function in later years. Blindness, mental deficiency, paralysis, deafness, abnormal permanent teeth begin to appear.

It is the duty of every pregnant woman to make sure that she is free from syphilis and that she stays free from syphilis. The USPHS recommends and most states require by law that doctors take a blood test as early as the pregnancy is detected, and again at the beginning of the last three months of pregnancy. These are simple enough procedures for patient and physician alike.

Blood Tests: The Serology of Syphilis

"Serology" means the study of the serum, that is, the study of the antibodies and immune factors that float around in the noncellular serum of the blood. Whereas with gonorrhea there are (almost) no immune factors known and no way to diagnose the disease with a blood test, with syphilis accurate blood tests have existed for 60 years. Present-day applications of two basic, simple, and quick tests have made it possible to diagnose correctly every person who has syphilis without missing anybody or including anybody who doesn't have it. Although the exact names of tests vary from lab to lab, two types of tests predominate.

The first type is exemplified by the VDRL test, a modification of the famous Wassermann test. It takes its name from the Venereal Disease Research Laboratory in Atlanta, Georgia, which for 50 years served as the front line of research in the venereal diseases. (Through a recent bureaucratic shuffling that left doctors gasping all over the country, the VDRL as a centralized research lab was disbanded in 1973.) The VDRL test is a qualitative nonspecific test; like other standard tests for syphilis (STS), it indicates the presence of antibody-like substances called "reagin" found in the blood of syphilis patients and also in blood of some patients with tuberculosis, malaria, cowpox, and chronic inflammatory diseases like rheumatoid arthritis, lupus erythematosus, and polyarteritis nodosa. The VDRL and other STS are negative ("nonreactive") in the incubation period, but usually become positive ("reactive") a week or two after the primary chancre develops. They are always positive by the time secondary and later stages arrive. If the VDRL is positive in the face of clear clinical symptoms of syphilis, the diagnosis can be confidently made. If the VDRL is positive when no symptoms exist, specific tests should be done to rule out a "biologic false positive."

Specific tests involve direct fixation of the syphilis germs in the blood with laboratory chemicals that allow them to be visually identified under a microscope. To rule out a falsely positive VDRL blood test in the face of some other cause than syphilis, a specific test must be done. The fluorescent treponemal antibody test attaches a fluorescent dye to the syphilis germ, and the diagnosis literally glows in the dark under the microscope. This test, called the FTA-ABS, can be used with the VDRL to achieve virtually 100 percent accuracy.

In addition, the VDRL is used on a quantitative basis. By diluting the patient's serum 1:1, 1:2, 1:4, 1:8, and so on, one can determine the concentration of the syphilis antibody in the blood and thus the level of activity of the syphilis germ. If you have ever had a positive VDRL, you can have repeat tests at regular intervals to determine whether your treatment has been effective: if the VDRL antibody concentrations in your serum drop, the treatment is shown to be succeeding.

How *You* Can Prevent Trouble For *Yourself*

Thus we have come the long way to a conclusion promised many paragraphs above: what kind of measures you should personally take over the long run to keep from getting syphilis. Obviously, you should keep on the lookout for telltale eruptions on your own skin and your sexual partner's skin. Using condoms during sex lowers the risk of infection, but not to the extent as with gonorrhea. Showering immediately after sex does the same. People seem to be reluctant to do either most of the time.

The most important thing to do is to have VDRL blood tests twice a year, every year, from now on. These tests are cheap, indeed free at many public health places, YMCAs, gyms, and public baths. Often you are given one automatically in your job situation or at regular health checkups. You should always know your status in this respect. If you get syphilis, return for quantitative follow-ups of the VDRL to make sure you have been cured. Your VDRL should return to negative eventually, if you discover the disease no later than the secondary stage of syphilis. If you discover the disease in a later stage, the VDRL test may not become negative, but should decrease to a weak positive reaction if you are cured. If, upon reading this, you recall having had something like primary and/or secondary syphilis some time ago and never bothered about it, *get yourself immediately to a doctor and have him do the test.*

Whether or not you have a lot of sex, and even if you assume that you and your regular sexual partner are the most faithful of couples, have a regular VDRL checkup twice a year. If you are a woman you should have an additional VDRL in your first month and your last three months of pregnancy. Syphilis should be regarded as a silent infection for the most part, for nowadays the kind that is never detected in youth will cause the greatest trouble later in life.

Treatment

Treatment consists of penicillin, penicillin, or penicillin. While resistance to penicillin by gonorrhea has become a nuisance, although not an insurmountable problem, there has been NO resistance to penicillin by the syphilis spirochete *in 30 years*. In people allergic to penicillin, oral erythromycin and tetracycline are the best alternate drugs, but closer follow-up care is required because the patient has to take doses four times daily for two weeks and the doctor cannot be sure that the patient will remember. Recent reports by Italian medical investigators indicate that ampicillin will soon be recommended also under *some* circumstances.

If a person is known to have been exposed to syphilis, but no clinical sign or positive blood test has had time to develop, the doctor should give a preventive dose of penicillin. (See Appendix B.) It is foolish to wait for something to develop, while the person can spread the disease to others.

Within 24 hours of adequate treatment, the person ceases to be infectious. Please be sure your doctor gives you the OK before you enter the swim of things again. It is also essential that you help the doctor eliminate all the syphilis germs in your own life and in others by helping him identify and treat all those with whom you have slept in the pertinent past. You should confide in your doctor and in the public health people and tell them with whom you have slept. Public health investigators are discreet. If your doctor fails to report your infection to them, he is NOT doing you a favor.

You will be promptly reinfected by your previous sexual partners and you may be consigning others to an awful fate. Such information is not used by police authorities but remains private to trained health workers. Most young people, who used to be reluctant to reveal names, now realize that the important thing is to treat the disease.

Exact dosages recommended by the USPHS CDC in Atlanta can be found in the treatment schedules for syphilis, reprinted *in toto* in Appendix B.

Prevention on a Collective Basis

The community as a whole, and public health services in particular, can do a lot to eradicate syphilis totally. It is a fact that China, with 800 million peasants, has totally eradicated gonorrhea and syphilis in the past 20 years. Their technology is exactly like ours, but their motivation and organization of public health workers are far more effective. We do not need to adopt a totalitarian authority to effect the same change in venereal health. Indeed the 350 federal public health workers who have been assigned to travel around the country tracking down cases and epidemics of syphilis have kept the rate of syphilis down even in the face of the current gonorrhea epidemic. If this understaffed crew were augmented four or five times, we could do much better. With increased reporting by physicians to the Public Health Service, with venereal disease education programs in schools for young people, with massive screenings of blood tests at clinics of non-venereal diseases and at jobs, the problem can be eradicated here as well.

Exactly how the program could be massively implemented can be left to expert epidemiologists and physicians. Basically, complete eradication would involve massive screening of every person on a regular basis. Every doctor in this country should give twice-annual VDRL blood tests to ALL his patients—whether he is in private practice, in a large firm's health department, giving routine insurance screenings, in gynecologic practice, or in teen-age acne specialization. There should be laws to this effect; but until there are—and let's face it, what congressman is going to vote to make his constituents have mandatory syphilis tests twice a year?—every doctor should do it on his own. And until every doctor does it, it's up to YOU. Mobilize yourself and your friends to get your own regular VDRL twice-yearly checkups. You can't save the rest of the country, but you can help yourself and those you love.

As far as getting rid of the disease in one massive bold stroke, it would take a vaccine given to everyone overnight, like the polio vaccines. As with gonorrhea, this dream is elusive, although, as we have indicated, the body's response to syphilis provides a sounder immune reaction than does its response to gonorrhea. Currently tests for vaccines are underway. Dr. James Miller of UCLA, for one, has been able to immunize rabbits against active virulent strains of syphilis and is working on the early stages of human testing. However, as with gonorrhea, since there is no long-lasting immunity in treated patients who have actually contracted the disease, there is obviously great difficulty in providing immunity to people who have not had the disease by rigging up some hypercombination of antibody proteins. Do not wait for these bluebirds to go over the rainbow; you have to make the effort yourself to get regular blood test checkups and seek diagnosis and treatment whenever necessary. Syphilis is not the terror it once was, but it is still too awful to ignore.

Chapter Six:

VIRUSES AND SEX

Introduction

How many times has a doctor looked at you sympathetically and shrugged, "It's just a virus that's going around"? There are viruses that make the rounds sexually, too, and though they affect diverse functions of the body, they have several things in common. First, viruses are smaller than bacteria; they affect the lymph glands and blood defenses throughout the body, swelling your lymph glands ("nodes") and making you feel pretty rotten all over. Second, viruses are more persistent than bacteria and tend to come on more gradually and fade away more slowly than bacteria. Third, and most important, there has yet to be a real "breakthrough" in the fight to cure viruses. Whereas antibacterial drugs such as penicillin and tetracycline are so specific and so effective that we now can afford to treat such dreaded diseases as syphilis nonchalantly, there isn't a single similar drug that kills viruses without killing off some of the patient as well. In other words, when your doctor tells you that you have got one of those viruses that are going around, he means you're going to have to live with it as best as you can. What the doctor can do for you—and what you must do for yourself—when fighting any virus is use the best supportive measures to enable your body's natural defenses to throw off the virus. The body's antiviral antibodies and white blood cells are sure fighters, but slow.

There may be one or two disease problems in this chapter you have had without having got them from lovemaking. All of the diseases in this chapter are *commonly* obtained by direct physical contact with the infectious agent in some way *other* than by having sex with someone. Nevertheless, it is important to know that these diseases are transmitted by sexual physical contact in numbers that are increasingly recognized more each day. Knowledge about sexual transmission of hepatitis, for instance, is just now hitting the medical journals for the first time.

Viral Hepatitis

What Is It?

"Hepatitis" means inflammation of the liver (*hepar,* liver; and *-itis,* inflammation). The name *viral hepatitis* refers to that sort of liver inflammation caused by the acquisition of a certain virus or viruses, as opposed, say, to the liver swelling caused by drinking excess alcohol over a long time or some poison over a short time, or by some infectious agent other than a virus. Since there is no specific cure for this infectious agent, you may guess that not much is known about it. You are right. Only recently has the actual virus responsible for this disease been demonstrated to the satisfaction of medical experts.

What is known is that there are two types of virus that, once acquired, cause the same type of liver disease. The virus of *infectious hepatitis* has some physical quality that enables it to survive gastric acidity after being swallowed and be absorbed, arriving at the liver in time to multiply, destroy liver cells, and cause disease. The virus of *serum hepatitis,* while causing the same disease pattern as that of infectious hepatitis, can only get to the liver by being injected into the flesh (and hence the bloodstream) by a needle or sharp instrument recently used by a person who is already developing hepatitis. *Infectious hepatitis* can *also* be transmitted by direct blood-to-needle-to-blood contact.

What this means is that the viruses of infectious hepatitis are excreted by the liver into the intestinal tract and make their way to the feces and thus to the outside world. Serum hepatitis viruses are most often *not* found in the lower intestinal tract and are *not* found in the feces or in anything contaminated from feces. If you know that, you can easily understand why the two types of hepatitis are acquired as they are. Epidemics of infectious hepatitis occur generally when there is a massive breakdown in the normal sanitary conditions of a crowded situation. In a dormitory, such as a military or recreational camp, toilet pipes that leak into the drinking water can transfer the virus from one infected person to all of his or her community within a short period of time. If a city lets its sewerage flow into a body of water where commercial shellfish fishing is done, epidemics of infectious hepatitis can hit a large number of raw-shellfish eaters in a very short time, before health authorities have a chance to remedy the situation. At a doctors' convention an epidemic of infectious hepatitis was caused by raw clams fished from the Hackensack River, some years ago. This kind of pollution, among others, prompted the citizens of that area to initiate a massive cleanup of that river, which is now much improved. Occasional cases of infectious hepatitis, as opposed to epidemics, may occur when the contaminated feces are adequately contained by sewerage and sanitary conditions. In this case, the virus does not make it big in disease circles and must settle for the small time: a relative here, a friend there, a schoolmate elsewhere. It is often easy to track down the source of epidemic hepatitis, but it is almost impossible to pinpoint the origin of scattered, individual cases.

Serum hepatitis and infectious hepatitis may both be transmitted by blood-to-blood contact. Unsterile needles are the primary vehicle of exchange; that is why heroin addicts who share needles, in their slow suicidal fraternity, have such a high rate of serum hepatitis. Blood transfusions to innocent ill people in hospitals have an alarmingly high rate of serum and infectious hepatitis virus transfer. Five patients out of a thousand who get blood transfusions develop jaundice (yellow body color) from hepatitis acquired from the transfusions; another 75 patients out of the thousand get the virus but show no effects from it. Most of these cases of transfusion hepatitis in hospitals can be traced to blood donated from centers where people sell their blood; a high percentage of people who sell their blood need the money for heroin and the like. Selling blood is a practice that should be stopped; get your blood from the Red Cross or a similar organization if you can.

What has all this to do with sex? You may well ask. As far as serum hepatitis goes, the answer is "nothing," unless you share needles with your bedmate. We are becoming aware that infectious hepatitis has as a major mode of spread the vehicle of sex. Any hepatitis virus from an infected person's lower intestinal tract that you swallow is likely to give you hepatitis. This means that *if you have oral-genital contact with a person with infectious hepatitis, you run a high risk of getting the disease yourself.* You do not have to have oral-anal contact; the entire anal and genital area is moist, and the virus survives nicely in the entire area. Fellatio, cunnilingus, or licking the groin will serve to transmit the virus, if it is there, as well. As these practices are very common today (and were yesterday, probably), sexual transmission of infectious hepatitis is very, very common.

When is the person with infectious hepatitis virus infectious to you? The most infectious period is that person's own incubation period, when he has no symptoms or when they are just beginning. In that period the viruses are present in his liver and intestinal system in the greatest numbers. They are shed through the feces and can infect someone else before the donor himself shows symptoms (if any) of the disease. By the time a person has turned yellow from hepatitis, he is shedding many fewer viruses and is much less infectious to others. On the other hand, by the time he has turned yellow, you wouldn't touch him with a 10-foot pole.

Symptoms

Anywhere from two weeks to six months after acquiring the infectious hepatitis virus, the patient may develop symptoms. You should know that your body's defenses may be adequate to fight the virus off even if it does reach your liver; in that case you will never know you had the disease, but you can still spread it to others. The symptoms are mild, if you look at the vast body of people who have had the infection. Those who do develop symptoms will abruptly get a flulike syndrome of fever, chills, and muscle and bone aches and pains all over. At first you will feel that you have the flu and it will pass in a day or two. It doesn't. You begin to feel as though you have been pounded with a sledgehammer all over your body. Terrible weakness and lethargy develop; getting out of bed even to go to the bathroom becomes a chore. Headache is common; you lose your appetite. Cigarettes and liquor become unthinkable; even the smell may nauseate you. Nausea, vomiting, and diarrhea may follow. Abdominal pain may occur, and a reddening of the skin and even a rash. The urine becomes granular and discolored with orange bile; the stool loses its color and seems a pale gray. Just when you think you're going to die, you begin to turn yellow and/or begin to feel better. The fever subsides, the appetite returns, and you slowly return to some interest in life, even while the yellowness (jaundice) gets worse for a while, and then subsides.

During this period the liver may be enlarged, swollen, and tender to the touch. The liver, as the regulator of the blood's defenses and metabolism, is, among other things, a large filter that is particularly affected by the virus in question.

Diagnosing Infectious Hepatitis

If you get these symptoms, you will undoubtedly go to a doctor who will make the diagnosis by obtaining blood samples and finding characteristic elevations of enzymes released by the hepatitis-damaged liver. Thus you will have the diagnosis within a day or two of going to the doctor. One blood test in particular—the

Australian antigen test—will tell you whether you have serum or infectious hepatitis.

Depending on the severity of the illness as it appears clinically and by lab tests, you may require hospitalization for several days or even weeks. *There is a wide range of effects from this disease; it may hit someone hard and someone else very lightly.* Absolute bed rest is always indicated for some period of time; you will have to have nursing care either in a hospital or at home from your family. Normal business cannot be conducted.

Taking the Cure

The only way to beat hepatitis is to give in to it completely. Do exactly what your doctor says. You will be plagued by incredible tiredness day after day and will soon become impatient with sitting in bed and watching "Let's Make a Deal" for three straight weeks. But if you decide you are your own doctor and get out of bed and go back to work prematurely, you may have recurrences of hepatitis in the future and run the risk of developing cirrhosis of the liver and permanent, severe damage. If you take care of yourself well the first time around, there won't be any other times.

You will probably be placed on a low-fat, high-protein, high-carbohydrate diet. Sleep all you need to sleep, even if it's 18 hours a day at first. Don't push your recovery; by doing so you only risk not getting well. Drink as many fluids as you wish, and eat regularly, making sure to satisfy your appetite. Stay away from alcohol and cigarettes totally; you won't want to get near them at first. Your doctor will tell you when you may safely resume alcohol consumption; usually, it is about three months after all the body's enzymes have returned to normal and you are back to where you were physically before the attack. The critical period for abstinence from all alcohol is the first few months; it does not extend for a year or two, as was previously thought. Ask your doctor.

You should refrain from any intimate physical contact with anyone during the prejaundice period and during jaundice and for two to four weeks thereafter. Obviously, this means no sex of any kind. It also means scrupulous cleanliness in the household where you live. Preferably, you should have your own set of eating and drinking utensils; paper plates and cups and plastic forks, knives, and spoons are ideal. You should have your own bathroom, and stick to it. If you have to share a bathroom, always wash your hands carefully when using it and leave your toothbrush and drinking cup in a separate place. The bathroom that is shared should be disinfected with standard strong cleaning fluids several times a week.

Members of your immediate household, especially children, should probably get shots of gamma globulin at once after learning of the diagnosis. It is not clear that this actually helps, but it makes for peace of mind. If your contacts wait more than three days after learning of your diagnosis before getting gamma globulin, they are too late for it to have any effect and might as well skip it.

These are the standard precautions that must be obeyed. Period. Other than that, do not become paranoid. Your family may enter your room, as the virus does not hang in the air waiting to bomb the next victim. Visitors are unwelcome during the first few weeks because they feel uncomfortable in your presence, especially if you have become chartreuse, and because you have no strength to receive them. *This message should be communicated by your family politely but firmly to misguided well-wishers.*

Should you tell sexual contacts about your unhappy station? Yes, in all cases, but for different reasons. Anyone with whom you have had oral-genital contact within the past week should be notified at once so that he or she can go to the doctor and get a protective shot of gamma globulin. Anyone you saw prior to the last couple of weeks should be notified when you get the chance so that he or she may know not to worry. It is too late for him to do anything other than wait and see if he gets it. Don't try to figure out who gave it to you; it may have been a clam, and if it was a person, he or she didn't do it on purpose.

Once you have had infectious hepatitis, *if you thoroughly recover from your own case and do not have a relapse,* you have immunity to infectious hepatitis for the rest of your life. (You can still get serum hepatitis, however; so stay away from needles.) Don't fight it if you get it. Relax, rest, reassess your life, and be thankful for the chance to contemplate your (orange) navel.

Infectious Mononucleosis ("Mono")

To the teen-ager, newly filled with the wonders of sexual hormones, infectious mononucleosis has a romantic buzz about it, rather like a dueling scar in Germany. It is called "the kissing disease" by acne-ridden gossips the world over, and it is usually giggled that people who French kiss are particularly susceptible. Although one strongly doubts that being sick in any way can be romantic, it is likely that the (presumed) virus of infectious mononucleosis *is* transmissible by kissing (as infectious hepatitis is *not*) and probably by oral-genital contact (as infectious hepatitis is also). *However, even with such direct contact there is a much lower risk of acquiring the disease than for infectious hepatitis.*

Like the virus of infectious hepatitis, the virus of mononucleosis attacks the so-called reticuloendothelial system of the body, which includes the lymph nodes, the liver, the spleen, and certain other lymph tissues in the body. Infectious mononucleosis characteristically attacks the throat and the lymph nodes around the throat and neck, whereas infectious hepatitis virus does not. In other respects, however, mononucleosis can mimic infectious hepatitis, causing generalized weakness and malaise, and even swelling of the liver and jaundice.

Symptoms

After acquiring the virus by mouth-to-mouth or oral-genital contact, the patient (usually under the age of 30) will wait through an incubation period of several days to several weeks before getting some nonspecific symptoms like weakness and a general blah feeling, followed by fever, sore throat, and very bad headaches. With a fever, most people who are developing mononucleosis will get to the doctor. The sore throat may be unusually severe or persistent, and there may be noticeably swollen "glands" around the throat and under the tongue area. (On examination a doctor will almost always find some of these swollen nodes in these patients, whether or not the patient notices them himself.) There may be a fine rash or reddening of the skin. If jaundice is present, that means the liver is significantly affected, and thus signs of liver distress—nausea, lack of appetite, discolored urine, clay-colored stool—may also be present. It is rare for infectious mononucleosis to show all these signs, however.

Diagnosis

If you have "mono," the doctor will make the diagnosis by finding the severe lymph swellings about the neck, by the sore throat, and by finding a positive reading on a specific blood test for mononucleosis called the *heterophil agglutination* test. In addition, he will follow your liver enzymes to see whether or not the virus has affected liver function. Your progress will be charted by clinical recovery and by following the strength of the heterophil agglutination test in follow-up samples.

Recovery

As with infectious hepatitis and in fact with most viral diseases, rest and supportive therapy are the only cures available. Analgesics for the pain of sore throat will be prescribed by your doctor, and sedation if necessary. If the inflammation of the lymph nodes is severe and/or painful, steroid anti-inflammatory drugs may be given. There is some danger of rupturing your spleen with this disease; so undue activity during the convalescent period is unwarranted. The period of bed rest may last for several weeks, depending on the severity of the original symptoms and complications—such as bacterial throat infection—that may follow the virus.

There is no need for isolation in most cases, and relatives may freely have access to your room. This virus is much less contagious than the virus of infectious hepatitis, and separate eating utensils or bathrooms are not required. Mouth-to-mouth contact and sexual contact are to be avoided for the period of bed rest.

There is really little need to apprise recent sexual partners that you have got "mono"; even with direct contact there is a low risk of contagion, and in any event there is no way to ward off the disease should it have been already gaining a foothold in someone else. There are no gamma globulin shots effective as prophylactic measures.

Herpes Simplex

Herpes simplex is the name of the virus that causes chronic recurrent fever blisters of the lips. Herpes simplex type 2, identical in many ways, can cause single and recurrent eruptions on the genitals, a condition known as *herpes genitalis.* If a fever blister can be annoying on the lips, it can be excruciating on the genitals. The virus is widely spread throughout the population, but some people seem to have better defenses against it than others. Although many people, if their blood is studied in a test, will show antibodies against these viruses, only a minority have recurring symptoms.

From direct physical contact, person to person, the virus apparently penetrates the skin and multiplies locally in that area. You can acquire the virus from direct genital-to-genital sexual intercourse with someone who has the blisters on his or her genitals. However, even if an uninfected person does have sex with an infected person, there is not much risk that he will get the symptoms at all, since most people have immunity to the virus. Whether or not you can get fever blisters on your lip from blisters on someone else's genitals, and vice versa, is not clear, but probably is so.

If you do acquire the virus, and if you are not immune, and if the virus does take hold, within a few days tiny grouped blisters will appear. In the sexual organs, blisters occur especially on the head of the penis, on the loose skin of the uncircumcised penis, around the outside female vulva, and in the inside vagina and cervix. These blisters rapidly ulcerate and develop red centers. Usually the small blisters coalesce and become irritated by constant rubbing and chafing in the crotch. Secondary bacterial infection often sets in, and pus or other drainage may develop. The symptoms begin with itching, and as the ulcers worsen, the pain may become so intense that the victim does not even wish to walk or move and may require sedatives. Urination may become painful because of swelling of the penis or irritation of the urine on the female vulva. Sexual intercourse becomes unthinkable.

The first time the patient develops these symptoms, he will undoubtedly not know what they mean and will rightly go to the doctor. The doctor must take blood tests and culture the drainage to distinguish the ulcers from those of syphilis, chancroid, and so on. In general, the pain of herpes simplex of the genitals is much worse than of the other ulcerating genital diseases except chancroid, but clinical impressions cannot be relied upon.

Therapy

Again, there is no specific cure. Soothing dressings and topical anesthetics and ointments may be required to alleviate severe inflammation, pain, and itching. Secondary bacterial infections (which are common) may require specific antibiotic therapy for the secondary bacteria. In severe recurrent cases certain cytotoxic drugs such as iododeoxyuridine may be applied. The groin should not remain moist or wet, or the skin will become macerated and secondary infection will surely set in. The patient must be instructed by the doctor how to keep the area dry yet not chafingly so.

Each initial attack and each recurrence generally subsides in two weeks or so, of its own natural course. In this time the body activates its own antibody system. The ulcers do not usually spread from one part of the body to another. *If you originally get herpes simplex on your lips, you will probably never have it on your genitals, and vice versa.*

Recurrences

Unfortunately, the herpes virus is never cleared totally from the body and remains latent at the site of original penetration of the skin. Precipitating factors—like pregnancy, menstruation, emotional strain, fever, common colds, other infection, gastrointestinal disturbances, and irritating foreign bodies or allergy-producing fabrics at the site in question—may cause the virus to multiply and cause symptoms anew. Abrasion or excessive friction to the groin may stimulate a recurrence in the previously afflicted person.

One consolation is that, possibly because of the acquisition of antibodies with time, people over 30 rarely get new cases of herpes simplex of the lips or the genitals.

Chapter Seven:
WARTS AND ALL

The words *syphilis* and *gonorrhea* are clinking fashionably off martini glasses at cocktail parties these days, like so many Noel Coward bons mots, but did you ever hear anybody talk about the three so-called "minor" venereal diseases, lymphogranuloma venereum, granuloma inguinale, and chancroid? These three diseases were all discovered about a century ago and have in common annoying, sometimes outrageous-looking skin lesions around the genitals and a propensity to turn up in tropical climates and on economically deprived people, especially blacks. With these three diseases, we group in this chapter also "venereal warts," which are viral warts caused by viruses not much different from those elsewhere on the body except that they grow, often in large ugly clusters, around the crotch. All four of these "minor" venereal diseases give annoying, sometimes secondarily infected skin problems; with the skin irritations of herpes simplex discussed in another chapter, they are the only venereal diseases to cause massive, unattractive, and really painful skin problems.

In other words, the diseases in this chapter cause wet, ugly, unaesthetic, smelly, repulsive warts, growths, and irritations of the skin around the genitals. Nobody likes to talk about them much, including doctors. Examining a patient with one of these problems who has let himself (herself) go can be a really ghastly experience. Because they are so unattractive, because many cases turn up in people who have poor standards of hygiene, and because often they are assumed to be "tropical" diseases, these disorders have been given the short end of the stick as far as medical attention goes. You still find experts arguing, in fact, whether these skin lesions are "venereal" or not, when clearly they are most often found on the genitals and most often transmitted by sexual contact. The old stereotype of the promiscuous black newly arrived from the Caribbean with these diseases no longer holds, however. There have been numerous cases reported among middle-class blacks and whites, and doubtless even more *unreported* cases among well-off classes. These diseases will remain "minor" in the sense that they are less prevalent and neither as infectious nor as dangerous as syphilis or gonorrhea; nowhere near the number of people in America will suffer from them as will suffer from the "major" venereal diseases or even from crabs. But as sexual and social mobility continues to cut across race, sex, and economic levels, these problems will appear in all segments of the population in more noticeable numbers than before. And people with the "minor" venereal diseases often have intense pain, debility, and itching that seem a lot more important than the often half-hearted symptoms of the "major" venereal diseases. There is no inherent racial preference with these diseases, although the organisms responsible for the skin lesions do seem to thrive in tropical climates. Whoever you are, you are more at risk if you are poor, or in a rundown state of health generally, or do not maintain good hygiene.

Venereal Warts

A wart is a wart is a wart. Warts are caused by viruses, and "venereal warts" are ordinary, harmless warts caused by city slicker viruses that prefer to concentrate around the genitals. Like other warts, they may come singly or in numbers and may go away by themselves. Venereal warts have adapted to life in the genital region and thus are commonly spread by sexual contact.

The chief problems of venereal warts—also called genital warts or *condylomata acuminata*—are three. First, they must be distinguished from the syphilitic warts of the secondary stage of syphilis, called *condylomata lata*. These two types are virtually indistinguishable in appearance. In other words, if you get a wart around your genitals, it is perfectly natural for you to wonder if that wart is innocent or if it indicates syphilis. You should of course see a doctor and let him find out scientifically. The second problem is that venereal warts tend to hang around a long time, ulcerate, become secondarily infected with bacteria, drain pus, smell, spread, and hurt a great deal. Needless to say, under those conditions, neither you nor a potential sexual partner will be much interested in having sex. The third problem is that these warts can spread to other people with genital contact.

Venereal warts are soft, pink, fleshy outgrowths on the skin around the external genitals and on the mucous membrane inside the genitals. In men they occur at the end of the penis around the foreskin or at the opening of the urethra. In men—not always homosexual men—they also occur around the anus. In women they are commonly seen on the external vulva and spread around to the anus. Beginning as tiny nondescript swellings, they grow quickly into clusters of long warts. They may fuse into a cauliflower-like tumor. If there is a coincidental vaginal discharge—as from *Trichomonas,* for instance—the warts grow very quickly and become macerated, painful, and smelly. They also grow on the inside vaginal wall and the cervix.

Venereal warts are *very* common. Most people clean themselves; so usually simple hygiene keeps the problem down to one or two innocent, painless, even unnoticed warts. It is only a small percentage of people in whom the warts begin to engulf the entire genital area and cause real misery. Men and women are at equal risk, and the warts are as worldwide as all other warts. People can also spread warts to themselves and to others by fingering the lesions and by unwitting hand contact, but this method of transfer is NOT a risk significant enough to bother yourself about.

Symptoms include irritation and/or itching that ranges from ho-hum to excruciating, depending on the extent of the lesion. Unfortunately placed warts about the anus may cause painful defecation or blood-tinged toilet tissue. Obviously, the larger the warts get and the more they spread, the more the impairment of sexual function and even walking, as the warts rub against the skin. Warts that grow into the urethra can cause urinary retention and urethral irritation.

RARELY, well-established, long-lasting venereal warts may undergo a change into a skin cancer. For the ordinary person engaged in any variety of sexual encounters, with or without a history of innocent venereal warts, this need not be a worry. For the person with chronic, gross, or neglected venereal warts of long standing, a biopsy may be indicated merely as a precaution. One hesitates even to mention the possibility of the development of cancer, because the word is such a terrifying one; it can be repeated that the risk is slight. Nevertheless, it should serve as a stimulus to get to the doctor as soon as you see the first wart.

Treatment

Spontaneously, venereal warts may disappear. Estimates for the possibility of such an occurrence range in the medical literature from 10 to 75 percent. It is well known that warts have a certain tenacity no matter where they occur; they are caused by viruses, and viruses are not as susceptible to medical treatment as are bacteria, which often give in after the first dose of antibiotic. Therefore, with the wide range of therapies your doctor may consider, you should resign yourself to at least several appointments and checkups and dosages. The patient can count on some combination of local chemical ointment application, such as tincture of podophyllin. Experts are unanimous in saying that only the physician should apply this ointment, as it can burn if incorrectly applied. No home remedies, please. There may be some need to use electrocautery (under local anesthetic) or, in gross cases such as those where the urethral outlet is obstructed, surgical excision. Some newer chemicals are being tested at the present time.

It is unfortunate that viruses have incomplete antibody-antigen reactions and are not subject to treatment by antibiotics as are bacteria. People simply have to put up with a little more inconvenience in getting rid of warts. Usually a few visits to the doctor will do, and any cautery or local surgery will be done under anesthetic, of course. Just remember that you minimize your risk by getting to the doctor as soon as you notice the first offending wart. First, you will need a blood test to make sure it isn't syphilis. Second, you can get rid of the venereal warts much easier when they first appear. Don't let false pride or embarrassment over the supposed unaesthetic appearance of your private parts keep you from seeing a doctor. Believe me, he has seen much worse. And part of the treatment will be a sincere reassurance that your problem has been diagnosed correctly, is being treated, and will go away.

Chancroid

Chancroid is to syphilis as Pepsi-Cola is to Coca-Cola; it ain't the real thing, but sometimes you need to read the label to be sure. It is a local disease and does not spread through the blood to destroy distant parts of the body, as syphilis does, but stays in and about the groin to cause local problems and local complications there. It is called "soft chancre," "soft sore," or "soft ulcer"; its causative agent is a bacillus (form of bacteria) discovered in 1889 by a man named Ducrey. Hence the responsible organism is called Ducrey's bacillus or *Hemophilus ducreyi.*

Symptoms

After contracting the organism from the genitals of a sexual partner, there is a three-to-eight-day incubation period before anything turns up. Then there is an ulcerated sore at the point of previous contact. It begins as an area of redness that blisters out and rapidly ulcerates. It becomes a smooth, round ulcer with a red, ragged margin and a small amount of pus draining from the center. *It looks very much like the primary ("hard") chancre of syphilis with one important but not always reliable exception: syphilis chancres do not hurt but chancroid sores hurt very much.* (There are no infallible rules in medicine, and occasionally the syphilis chancre can get secondarily infected by other bacteria and hurt like the dickens, but most of the time this rule is helpfully accurate.)

Men turn up with chancroid much more often than do women, possibly because it is harder to find the chancroid sore in the female anatomy. It is prevalent in all races, more common in the city than in the country; it is endemic in tropical and subtropical countries. Dr. William Brown, former chief of the CDC VD section in Atlanta, says, "Although accidental infections among physicians and midwives have been recorded, transmission is almost exclusively by sexual intercourse. Indiscriminate promiscuity and poor personal hygiene favor transmission."

In men the chancroid sores usually turn up at the end of the shaft of the penis, on or about the area of the foreskin. Other sexual areas such as the anus, scrotum, thighs, and even occasionally the hands and the mouth can be affected in both sexes. In women, ulceration is most common around the external vulva, around the urinary outlet. Vaginal or anal ulceration is less common.

Complications

Like any other invading organism, the Ducrey bacillus meets resistance as it tries to make its way through the skin into the body. The lymph-collecting systems tend to drain the organisms into the lymph nodes in the groin. Here a fierce battle ensues as white cells try to stave off the invasion, and the nodes swell, forming a painful and tender enlargement that is known as a *bubo.* (Any infected lymph node is known as a bubo, including the ones that give the name to bubonic plague, which is of course an entirely different disease.) As a result of all this microscopic warfare, large abscesses may form in the groin that can break through the skin and drain pus, as buboes of all kinds are known to do. Abscess formation in the groin occurs in about *half* the *untreated* cases. With abscess formation comes fever and general malaise. If a groin abscess forms, usually the skin lesions persist. They may also merge and begin to extend over the genitals, causing severe disfigurement of the genitals in a short time. These severe complications occur in less than half the untreated cases. Most cases are too painful to ignore, and treatment is available to all today.

Diagnosis

Your doctor will avail himself of some combination of microscopic examination of a smear from the ulcer or the pus, a culture of that material, or a biopsy. In addition, microscopic examinations for syphilis bacteria and syphilis blood tests should be done to make certain you don't have syphilis. And there are specific tests to do to exclude lymphogranuloma venereum and granuloma inguinale. Of all these diseases, if you had your choice, chancroid is the one to get.

Treatment

"With the advent of sulfonamides . . . the first therapy specific for any of the venereal infections was discovered. Sulfa drugs are still the treatment of choice for chancroid, although [other drugs] are also effective."

(Dr. Brown again.) Sulfonamides are given orally, not locally, and your doctor may direct you to give some special cleansing attention to the involved area. If lymph nodes have become affected, they must be drained as well. Remember that chancroid's complications are local and affect only the outside and inside genitals and the lymph nodes that drain the area. There are no blood tests or body-wide follow-ups needed. Treatment will be given for 10 to 14 days, and sexual contacts of yours must also be examined by the doctor and treated if necessary. Refrain from sex during treatment or until your doctor gives the all clear, whichever comes later.

Granuloma Inguinale

A "granuloma" is an excessive growth of scar formation indicating some disruption of the tissue by an invading live organism or an inert foreign particle. "Inguinale" refers to the groin. Whereas chancroid may content itself with one or two small ulcers, granuloma inguinale almost always continues to form new reactive growth and obliterative scar tissue locally over the groin in response to invasion by a peculiar bacteria known as the Donovan body (discovered by you-guessed-it in 1905). *Donovania granulomatis* is the formal name for the causative organism. The very nature of the disease, as indicated by its name, implies continuous scarring and obliteration of normal skin tissue. For this reason, this disease is not self-limited but progressive.

Reputable medical textbooks continue to say that this

disease is more common among poor people of both sexes and all races.

Symptoms

Early on, blisters appear, usually in groups, and quickly ulcerate. They may look like any other genital venereal disease at first, but they develop a heaped-up, exaggerated, fleshy elevated mass about the ulcers that hints at the granulomatous nature of the disorder. These grainy ulcers spread by direct continuity and take on a beefy red look. Contact with adjacent areas of the thigh or buttocks spreads the ulcers directly. For the most part, *these ulcers are painless.* Occasionally infection spreads sexually to the mouth or lips. The initial lesions are so small and painless that they are ignored, especially in women. But they do NOT go away, but insidiously spread to form granular ulcers about the genital and anal region. There are no lymph node buboes with this disease. Although the destructive scar tissue remains locally in the groin, untreated this disease can cause generalized weakness and a miserable existence. Before the days of antibiotics the prognosis was pretty grim, if not as terrifying as for some other diseases.

Diagnosis

By the time the patient gets to the doctor, the lesions have taken on a characteristic granulomatous appearance that makes clinical judgment alone pretty accurate. Donovan bodies can be demonstrated microscopically from small biopsies or smears.

Treatment

Because of the chronic, smoldering nature of the disease, treatment will not be instantaneous. Various antibiotics are currently in use that require oral administration; no local preparations are smeared on the affected areas. Long-entrenched cases are hard to eradicate, however, and as with almost every disease in the history of mankind, the earlier you get medical attention, the more likely you are to get rid of the problem. Once anatomical destruction is effected, it is permanent.

There is still a great deal of controversy as to whether this disease is transmitted by sexual contact, but most doctors still believe it is; it would seem wise to refrain from sex after the diagnosis is made, at least through the first stages of therapy. Ask your own physician.

Lymphogranuloma Venereum

If you wonder why all the names of diseases in this chapter are so confusingly overlapped and redundant, it is because when the diseases were "discovered" they were poorly understood and therefore fuzzily named. Unfortunately, the story with lymphogranuloma venereum is still confusing. This disease is also called lymphopathia venereum, climatic bubo, tropical bubo, and one other name so similar to the disease we just finished that I dare not mention it for fear of having you throw up your arms in defeat. The causative agent is a *chlamydia* organism that is said to be "somewhere between a virus and a bacterium" until they find out what the heck it really is.

Symptoms

After a widely variable incubation period (a few days to several months), a small blister may appear at the site of sexual contact with the organism. Far more than with other venereal diseases, however, this blister is unnoticed and disappears without having been observed. It is rarely, if ever, found in women. The organism quickly makes its way to the inguinal lymph nodes and causes a bubo, or swelling in the lymph nodes. Pain is usually the first symptom noticed; the victim becomes aware of tender swelling in the groin. The nodes may spontaneously drain to the surface of the skin. Chills, fever, and general malaise may accompany the bubo, but these constitutional symptoms may be absent. If left untreated, the infection usually spreads to all the lymph nodes in the groin and thigh, although the body's defenses may be adequate enough to heal spontaneously within a few weeks. If the problem is allowed to become chronic, many swollen buboes may burden the entire area, with a backup of lymph fluid resulting in engorgement of the lymph-collecting system. This backup of lymph fluid in the tissues causes grotesque swelling of the penis, female vulva, or thighs that is one kind of *elephantiasis*. In addition, secondary skin changes about the penis or vulva may occur, with discolorations, ulcerations, or warty outgrowths. These are long-term consequences of lack of treatment and take months to develop. At any stage the whole process may come to a halt, either temporarily or permanently.

Complications

As a late complication of the destructive process, urinary, genital, and rectal function deteriorates. Elephantoid growths hideous to behold distort the vulva, the penis, or the anus. Because of poor lymph drainage of the tissues, an obstruction may encircle the rectum, making passage of stool painful and difficult. Swollen rectal linings can bleed and cause great pain. Once these strictures occur, they can be ameliorated only by surgical dilatation. Urethral ulcerations also occur. As a final insult, the lesions of lymphogranuloma venereum can undergo malignant change to skin cancer.

These complications are not inevitable; even untreated the process varies widely from one patient to the next.

Diagnosis

There is a specific skin test like the TB test in which a lymphogranuloma venereum (LGV) antigen is injected and the skin reaction read at 48 and 72 hours. In addition, the organism can be obtained from a bubo and cultured for identification.

Therapy

There are a number of antibiotic agents given orally that arrest the organism and stop its destructive anatomical changes. Once anatomical damage has been done, surgical intervention may be required. Moral: get to your doctor early.

Summary

These diseases can be among the most alarming in medicine; they are most unaesthetic and even humiliating to the sufferer. Ironically, although they look so awful, they are less dangerous than insidious diseases like syphilis and gonorrhea, which can cause damage throughout the whole person. A fair percentage of those reading this book can expect to have an innocent venereal wart or two, with little or no cosmetic or anatomical damage. The other diseases are much more rare, but on the increase in today's sex-charged society. You do not need to be a poor person or a black to get these diseases; you do not need to be a homosexual to get rectal strictures from lymphogranuloma venereum; nor do you need to expect the worst if you should acquire one of these diseases. The best—the only—thing to do is to go straight to the doctor the first time a suspicious skin lesion, wart, outgrowth, pimple, blister, lump, sore, or elevated area appears anywhere in your groin, painless or painful. Do not play Dr. Gillespie, diagnostician. Whatever the correct diagnosis, you will save yourself a lot of worry and bother by getting immediate medical attention.

Chapter Eight:

DILDOES, DOUCHES, AND DOODADS: Are You Getting Any Friction?

Sex means friction of one sort or another, and like anything else it can be too much or too little of a good thing. There is a wide range of trouble you can get into because of excess friction resulting from sexual activity. "Excess" is here a relative word; what's good for the gander may not be good for the goose. The same sexual activity that may cause abrasion, soreness, and bladder infection in a previously virginal girl may be only a tease for a platinum-haired matronly swinger from Long Island.

The natural integrity of skin and internal membrane surfaces must be preserved in the body as a whole if good health is to be preserved. This integrity, the single most important defense we have against foreign intruders like bacteria, is compromised by the friction of sex, and germs can penetrate the "wounded" skin and take hold. The natural lubrication of the vagina and the pubic hair protects against abrasion and infection as well. All these defenses must be preserved if the sexual parts are to stay healthy. Too much douching removes the natural lubricant of vaginal secretions and leaves the vagina more susceptible to injury and infection. The trick is to learn how to roll with the punches in order to maintain the natural delicate balance of surface and internal integrity of the sexual and urinary organs. This chapter describes a number of problems arising from different frictional irritations of the sexual parts, and ways to solve them.

Honeymoon Cystitis

Cystitis means infection of the bladder; "honeymoon cystitis" arises, generally in women, after a period of sexual intercourse in a previously virginal person. The mechanism is simple; because of repeated pneumatic and frictional insult to the inner organs, the opening of the urethra is irritated, and germs travel back up the urethra to the bladder, causing an infection there. The condition is far more common in women because the urethral outlet is at the outlet of the vagina and can easily be irritated by the penis. The female urethra is much shorter than the male urethra, and germs have less distance to travel to get back up to the bladder. (Incidentally, the urine and the bladder are always absolutely sterile in the healthy person, and any infection or bacterial contamination of the bladder means something is going wrong. It is incorrect to think of normal urine as "dirty." The feces are loaded with bacteria, but the urine normally does not contain a single bacterium.)

A few days after repeated sexual intercourse in the person who will develop cystitis, the sufferer will begin to feel an uncomfortable sensation about the bladder. Urination will be more frequent and uncomfortable, perhaps "itchy." There will be a spastic, uncontrollable quality to urination, and even pain on urination. The urine may discolor slightly or actually develop pus. In any event, the person will be uncomfortable enough to see a doctor. Episodes of honeymoon cystitis can be easily treated with common antibacterial agents. The organisms involved are *not* the bacteria of syphilis or gonorrhea, but common, usually harmless bacteria that populate the normal vulva or penis exterior and are simply pushed away from their normal location up the urethra to the bladder.

Bladder infections are not to be treated lightly, however, because the infection can travel farther up the urinary tract and attack the kidneys themslves. Kidney infections are very serious indeed. Don't let the infection get that far: if you have an itchy, spastic, spurty urination after episodes of sexual intercourse that until recently was unusual for you, get to a doctor.

A Principle of Hygiene

Honeymoon cystitis illustrates an important point in personal hygiene. Since bacteria can travel from where they do no harm to where they can cause trouble, one objective in keeping clean should be to keep bacteria away from where they should not be. In women, care must be routine to keep fecal contamination away from the vulva and vagina. Tissue paper used after bowel movements should be wiped from the anus posteriorward, away from the front of the body and the vagina. Tissues used after urination should not be rubbed back and forth, but with one clean stroke should be wiped away from the external vulva and not back to it. The idea is to go from the least bacterially populated part to the more populated part, and not back again.

Bartholin Gland Abscesses

Bartholin glands are small normal glands located immediately behind the labia majora (outer lips) of the vulva. Their glandular secretions supply natural lubrication to the vagina, which lies posterior to the glands. They are part of the normal system of lubrication and surface integrity that frames this chapter. Since the glands are dead-end spaces with the only outlet to the outside, they are subject to retrograde invasion by normal skin bacteria. The friction of sex or of normal manipulation can sometimes force bacteria up into the gland openings and back to the glands themselves. In these cases, infection sets in. The glands swell up to the size of grapes or even larger, become extremely painful to the touch, redden, and may drain pus. Since there is one Bartholin gland on each side of the vulva, these swellings may occur on one side or on both sides of the labia majora. Fever and general malaise may develop, and sexual intercourse becomes unthinkable; urination may aggravate the painful sensation. In all cases a doctor will be seen. The treatment is to clean and drain the involved area and administer appropriate general antibiotics. After appropriate therapy, further complications do not ensue, and the affected area returns to its normal configuration and painlessness. Bartholin gland infections are not common, but are not rare, either. Infections of Bartholin's glands are not transmitted from one sexual partner to the other.

Hemorrhoids

Hemorrhoids are abnormally distended, swollen varicose veins just inside the anus and in the lower rectum. They cause severe pain on defecation or when any pressure is put upon them and frequently are associated with bleeding and infection. Sexual intercourse, especially rectal intercourse, can cause excruciating pain in a person with hemorrhoids. Hemorrhoids are worse in people who have irregular bowel habits or undue exertion of the bowels from nervous tension, constipation, diarrhea, or pregnancy. They are most common around the age of 40.

Hemorrhoids may cause no problems in some cases. If there is only minor difficulty, sterile lubricants for rectal and for vaginal intercourse can alleviate the situation. If hemorrhoids are severe, the patient should see a doctor for many reasons. Treatment of hemorrhoids may be conservative, with medication; it may be an office procedure, as in the new technique of cryotherapy (instant freezing) pioneered in this country by Dr. Howard J. Eddy of New York State; or it may be a full surgical procedure, with total excision of the offending varicosities. It should be noted that rectal infections such as from gonorrhea can aggravate preexisting but quiescent hemorrhoids and cause them to be symptomatic. Once again, it pays to keep on the alert to prevent these conditions from reinforcing each other.

Pilonidal Sinus Disease

A very common disorder in young people, and especially in young men during puberty and in their twenties, is the problem known as pilonidal sinus disease. "Pilonidal" means "a nest of hairs," and that is exactly what the trouble comes from: a burrowing of stray body hairs into a "nest" at the crease or dimple of the two buttocks. It is thought that the coarse pubic hairs of the crotch and the stubby hairs that fall down the back of the neck during a haircut come to rest in this dimple. There they are caught and constantly rubbed into the skin by the motion of the buttocks in sitting and walking. Irritation and redness of the skin develop, and the hairs actually burrow into the skin like a drill. Normal skin bacteria are introduced into the tissues, and an infection sets in. The infection may result in pus formation and a closed abscess; or the irritation and infection may not progress to this extent, and a less bothersome, more chronic irritation can set in.

In either case, the condition causes extreme pain upon sitting down, especially in a moving vehicle, and also during defecation and sexual intercourse, either vaginal or rectal intercourse. (The condition has caused thousands of sick days in the armed services and is known as "jeep driver's disease" in military jargon.) The sufferer will know that the exquisite tenderness he feels in these situations is far in excess of what those stresses should bring, and he will find on inspection a red and tender area at the base of his spine at the buttocks' crease. There may be a sinus tract or opening from within the skin that drains pus. In the case of an abscess, the whole area is swollen and extremely painful to the touch from the pus pocket trapped inside.

In most cases of chronic irritation with abscess formation or the presence of pus, conservative treatment clears the problem up. Careful and gentle cleansing of the area with soap and water should be done. Attention to sitting posture and the use of pillows to sit on alleviate the pressure and give the irritation a chance to heal. Showers should be taken after haircuts and regular daily hygiene maintained. Acute cases of abscess or pus formation can be managed by surgical incision of the area and drainage. Only in extreme cases is total excision of the area by a surgeon necessary.

Many people who have never heard of this disease will recognize some of the irritations from their own experience and should consult a doctor if the condition recurs. The condition usually flares up for a few months and then somehow goes into remission, unless an abscess forms in the meanwhile. There are few recurrences after the age of 30.

Dildoes and Other Substitutes

Anything that is longer than it is wide may be called a phallic symbol, and anything that is even the least bit concave may be called a vaginal symbol. Surely the history of psychiatry is replete with such assumptions; we have Freud's lighthouse and the flying penis of Leonardo da Vinci as examples, not to mention men's ties, Coca-Cola bottles (the art form of the century!), the Bankhead tunnel, figs, Cinderella's slipper, Joan Crawford open-toed sling-back pumps, and so on.

Dido and Aeneas made love as lightning flashed about her cave. Not surprisingly, phallic symbols often emerge from mere fantasy or figure of speech and are taken literally, used instead of the real thing. Some would argue that we are living in the Age of Dildoes. Surely they are all about us: one sees advertisements for "personal vibrators" even in the *New York Times* that seem shaped remarkably for vaginal use. Dildoes made in the exact shape of penises, in varying sizes and textures of rubber, are sold by mail and in so-called sextiques in our major Sodoms and Gomorrahs. Indeed Coca-Cola bottles provide more than one refreshing pause.

Are dildoes dangerous? In some cases yes, and in some no. Private dildoes you don't share with anyone else do not, at least, spread germs; you cannot give anything you already have to yourself. On the other hand personal dildoes should NOT be used in both the rectum and the vagina. The vagina is NOT dirty, but the rectum most certainly is; and infection can be introduced into the vagina from the fecal bacteria if dildoes are used in both places. Dildoes that are shared by two or more people at the same time, or in group sex, or even at different times, can spread all the diseases we have mentioned in this book. On the other hand, if you have sex with one person or more than one at the same time, you will probably come into direct contact with any germs that may be present, and the use of a dildoe will not increase this risk.

Vaginal use of dildoes can be well regulated; that is, there are exquisitely sensitive nerves in the vagina that tell a woman very quickly whether or not the dildoe is causing any mechanical difficulty or pain. Severe overstimulation with dildoes can cause abrasions and soreness, and abraded locations may become infected secondarily by bacteria.

One the other hand, rectal use of dildoes is another

matter. The inner part of the rectum is totally devoid of all the nerves we usually associate with the surface of the skin or of the vagina. There are no nerve endings anywhere in the intestines (which include the rectum) to sense pain, or heat, or a tear, or, for that matter, pleasure. The external skin about the anus is the only matter in rectal intercourse that feels anything. Anything else you feel during rectal intercourse is purely psychological. Thus if you insert a dildoe or anything else into the rectum, you run the risk of damaging the intestines without feeling the damage or having any clue about it until blood starts leaking out of your anus. Small dildoes gently applied by yourself may be harmless, but large ones may cause tears in the delicate intestinal membranes that result in peritonitis, severe hemorrhage, and other grave consequences. Usually the insertion of the penis into the rectum does not cause these problems because the penis does not come into contact with the internal intestinal wall and all sensation of friction is delivered by the outside anus skin. Large dildoes and other foreign objects—particularly those with edges or sharp points—must be prohibited. A friend of mine who was a general medical officer at a naval base once had to remove a candelabra from the vagina of a woman whose husband was away in Vietnam. When using substitutes, make the substitute as like the real thing as possible.

In moments of unbridled sadomasochistic passion, fists and even feet have been used as weapons of intercourse vaginally and rectally in both sexes. Such practice is extremely dangerous, especially in the rectum, where severe damage can be done to the intestinal membranes, resulting in hemorrhage and/or peritonitis. Although there is undeniably some component of forceful intrusion and pleasurable fulfillment in every kind of sexual intercourse, from a medical viewpoint—all "moral" prejudices aside—the use of fists and arms and man-made objects of large or sharp or unsuited size for intercourse can be clearly condemned. Moreover, fist fucking and the like constitute assault and mayhem in courts of law, even if the recipient at first consents.

Dildoes of one kind or another are very common and are used by all segments of society. The safest ones to use are those in the shape of penises and made of *pliant* rubber. Leave the Coca-Cola bottle to its intended purpose.

Douches

Somewhere back in the Neanderthal days of civilization the female sex was sold a bill of goods that the vagina was a dirty place especially during and after menstruation. Primitive rites, such as total body immersions in clear streams and douching, were developed to "cleanse" the female body. Such folklore, amazingly, remains nearly unchanged today, passed on explicitly and implicitly from mother to daughter, generation after generation. The fact of the matter is that the vagina is perfectly capable of maintaining a dynamic state of hormonal and hygienic balance. Its secretions and the anatomical tendency of the vagina to drain with gravity work to keep this most intimate of the female parts "clean" at all times unless some disease intrudes. Nevertheless, the myth of "dirtiness" is stamped on the impressionable mind of young girls and remains there, to be passed on to the next generation. The attitude, moreover, is deliberately perpetuated by selfish commercial interests that have much to gain from the sale of vaginal douche instruments and solutions. Advertising campaigns less than subtly suggest that marital and sexual difficulties may arise from vaginal "bad breath" and that a quick douche with such-and-such will solve not only this "embarrassment" but all sexual problems at once. Now in addition, within the space of two years, clever advertising men have created from nothing an industry of "feminine hygiene deodorants" without which, we are told, not even the cutest chick at Malibu will be able to get a man. The new "feminine hygiene sprays" are in effect the jet age douches, the aerosol bidets of the swinging seventies for the modern woman. Over 200 million dollars annually is already being spent on these sad testimonies to the perpetuated insecurities of women!

The fact is that all douches and vaginal deodorants are unnecessary, with very few exceptions. Indeed there are serious complications that may follow douching, such as peritonitis, and minor allergic reactions are not uncommon after using the female vaginal deodorants. The term *feminine hygiene* itself is a loaded argument that falsely assumes that the female body is not clean without some sort of extraordinary intervention, such as douching, by the owner of that body. "Feminine hygiene" is a precious put-down and an insulting term that should be abandoned at once.

The normal vagina has an acid pH of about 5.0 that is maintained by the nature of the secretions from the walls of the vagina. In a normal vagina, these secretions are not copious and do not cause any itch. There should be no noticeable secretion from the vagina to the outside of the body except for clear-colored "moistness" in the normal woman. (Periods of menstruation obviously involve a good deal of flow from the vagina.) Any woman who bathes regularly should not have any noticeable odor about the external female vulva; most "female" odors in the normal woman are due to dried urine on the pubic hairs, which builds up after 8 or 10 hours after urination. Daily bathing precludes such odor buildup, as it would for the male counterpart of such a problem. *If a woman knows she bathes regularly and yet has any significant vaginal odor or itch or discharge, she must assume that something is going wrong and she should see a doctor at once.* Many women, prejudiced by well-intentioned but wrong training from their mothers, assume that discharges and/or itches and/or odors are the natural curses of being a woman, and they shrug their shoulders resignedly and turn to the douche instead of the doctor. *Douching cannot cure any of the causes of itch or discharge or odor, although it can temporarily relieve the symptoms, thus masking the real problem and delaying its cure.*

In addition to the general inefficacy of douching to give real help to any significant disease problem, and beyond its superfluity in maintaining normal cleanliness, douching can cause specific dangers. First there is the matter of the danger of particular solutions used as douches. It is not uncommon in this country to use Lysol or a similar cresol solution for douching, although the thought makes one shudder. Lysol is the first cousin to carbolic acid, which may be fine on formica and stainless steel but can only be considered a poison when used on the skin or in a body cavity, like the vagina. Using Lysol to kill germs inside the body is like using an atom bomb to kill a fly. Under no condition should Lysol or any of the common household disinfectants or cleansers be used anywhere on or in the body.

Certain other toxic solutions are still used, carried on by the grapevine, for douching. These include heavy metal solutions like mercury bichloride, bismuth, and even arsenic. These horrible remedies are a leftover of the period of 70 years ago when medicine, flailing around in the dark for some treatment for syphilis, discovered that heavy metals kill the syphilis germ. They also kill the patient. *In no case should any substance containing any of these metals be used in or on the body, and the safest procedure to follow is not to use any solution for a douche unless it is prescribed by a physician.*

In addition, most of the devices used for giving douches are dangerous. The typical bulb squeeze syringe and other pressure devices for forcing liquids into the vagina are dangerous. Remember that there is a direct, though tortuous, connection between the outside world and the inside of the abdominal cavity of the female. Any material—air or liquid—getting into the vagina can wind its way through the cervix, along the uterine wall, through the oviducts, and emerge at the ovary into the abdominal cavity. If liquids are forced into the vagina, the risk of forcing them clear through to the abdomen is increased. A number of cases have been reported in the medical literature in recent years of peritonitis induced by force-squeezed douche solutions. Although the risk is slight, most gynecology experts for many years have advocated *not* using pressure douche devices in any case. The only acceptable douche method is the gentler one of a modified (and clean) enema bag hung about a foot higher than the vagina and with a simple vaginal nozzle. No squeeze bulb or pressure cuff should be used.

Douching is ineffective in preventing conception or stopping the spread of any of the venereal diseases. The reason is largely that douching does not last very long, and the fluid put into the vagina does not stay there long enough to kill germs or impede the quick sperm cell. Vaginal jellies and spermicides, which remain in the vagina for several hours, as directed, are much more effective for both these purposes, although they are not 100 percent foolproof.

Douching removes the natural lubricants of body secretions and kills off the normal bacterial flora that protect the vagina from more dangerous bacterial and fungal intruders. The quickest way to invite disease-producing bacteria is to kill off the friendly bacteria that were holding the fort before.

What good, then, is douching? In some cases of *Candida albicans,* of *Trichomonas* infections, or of abnormal nonspecific vulvitis or vaginitis in which a doctor has excluded the possibility of an infection, symptomatic relief—but NOT cure—can be effected by douching as directed by your doctor. *Routine douching is wrong,* no matter what your mother or that silly movie the boys in your fifth-grade class couldn't see said. Most doctors have wrongly resigned themselves to the well-established practice of douching and simply try to keep their patients from doing it to excess or from using toxic agents. But the correct attitude should be that douching should NOT be done at all unless a doctor prescribes it. And if any symptom arises—especially a discharge, itch, or "odor"—you should NOT douche but should see a doctor. And don't douche out of "modesty" before you see the doctor! He should be allowed to observe the exact condition that bothers you.

In no case should douching be relied upon for prevention of one of the venereal diseases or for prevention of pregnancy. It just doesn't work. And as far as the sale of douche bulb syringes and pressure douche devices and "feminine hygiene" sprays, if Ralph Nader has any spare time, he should look into them.

Vaginal Jellies and Creams

Although Mother Nature has provided natural juices for the penis and vagina to accommodate the proper balance of smoothness and friction, vaginal jellies have a useful role in sexual intercourse. First, the contraceptive jellies are remarkably effective in preventing the venereal diseases and in preventing conception, if used as directed. Usually the jellies must be left in the vagina for several hours after sexual intercourse to be effective. They are vastly superior to douching in both these respects and have little risk attached. Occasionally a person may develop an allergic or chemical irritation to vaginal jellies. In such cases, use of the jelly should be stopped and a physician consulted.

Rectal Lubricants

Rectal intercourse should always be accompanied by liberal use of some surgical-quality sterile lubricant. The rectum has no provisions for pneumatic friction from an external source, and the lubrication has to be supplied in order to avoid damage to the anus or rectum. Surgical lubricants are sold without prescription at all drugstores. Examples are Surgilube, K-Y, H-R, and so forth.

Rectal "Douching"

The rectum is clear of fecal material except during the act of defecation. Nevertheless, the surfaces of the rectal membranes may not be clean enough if sexual rectal intercourse is intended. "Douching" of the rectum can be easily achieved with common enema techniques, as with the use of Fleet's enema, which contains a plastic squeeze bottle and a harmless fluid solution that stimulates elimination of any fecal material in the rectum or lowest part of the intestine. Small enema bags or pliant plastic squeeze bottles may be filled with tap water at body temperature or thereabout, and the solution gently infused into the rectum, held for a few seconds, and released. Excessive pressure or overlong retention, as with all enemas, is dangerous and should be avoided at all costs. Do not use soapy or salty solutions or any solutions other than commercially prepared enema solutions or plain tap water. Other solutions might contain chemicals harmful to the intestinal membranes. Excessive use of enemas is to be avoided.

Chapter Nine: QUESTIONS AND ANSWERS

Q *Can pain during sex mean venereal disease?*

A Pain during intercourse, called "dyspareunia" officially, can mean a lot of things, including venereal infection, nonvenereal infection, ovarian and/or uterine tumors, or anatomically distorted internal organs. Pain during intercourse can also suggest a psychological problem. In all cases you should see a doctor about it.

Q *What about pregnancy and VD?*

A Pregnancy does not increase the likelihood of getting VD, but if a pregnant woman has syphilis or gonorrhea, the result can be a disaster for the baby. All pregnant women should have a blood test for syphilis at the beginning and end of their pregnancies and should be examined for the possibility of gonorrhea.

Q *How much vaginal odor is normal, and how much means something is wrong, like VD?*

A The question of "odor" is highly subjective, but in

most cases it is fair to say that with a really significant vaginal odor and/or discharge, something is wrong and a doctor should be consulted. Vaginal odors, even with discharges, do not necessarily mean infection. Similiar irritation can occur from other causes, such as IUDs (intrauterine devices against conception), vaginal tampons, irritating undergarments, and so on. Obese women tend to have more exocrine glandular secretions in the groin area that can be mistaken for vaginal secretions. In addition, it should be noted that most cases of venereal infection in women occur *without* any symptoms such as odor.

Q *Can gonorrhea germs spread from a man's rectum to his penis, and vice versa?*

A No, not without a middleman, or a middlewoman.

Q *Can gonorrhea germs spread from a woman's vagina to her own rectum?*

A Yes, but it does not happen in most cases. When a woman has rectal gonorrhea, it means she has had rectal intercourse until proven otherwise.

Q *Can you spread venereal warts (simple genital warts from viruses, nonsyphilitic ones) from the genitals to the hands?*

A No.

Q *Do genital fever blisters (herpes genitalis) spread to a person's own lips, and vice versa?*

A No.

Q *If you have a sore or some abrasion on your vulva or penis, does this always mean an infection?*

A No. Mechanical friction can cause sores and painful abrasions, even from masturbation. That is one reason you should see a doctor if you are in doubt; after the possibility of venereal infection has been eliminated, the sore may be safely attributed to mechanical irritation.

Q *Do you feel the anal chancres of syphilis?*

A Almost all forms of venereal disease go unnoticed in the rectum. In other words, you feel nothing at all, or very little. There may be some slight discomfort or streaking of blood on toilet paper. Rectal syphilis is undoubtedly a "hidden" reservoir that has had little medical attention until recently.

Q *How common are skin rashes and irritations in venereal disease?*

A Very common. Almost all venereal diseases cause some irritation of the skin. Dermatologists spend a lot of time figuring out whether a wide variety of skin disorders they see are due to the venereal diseases, especially syphilis. Irritations of the skin may take on many guises, from simple blisters that look like "pimples" to gross discoloration of the entire skin. Gonorrhea also causes a dermatitis (irritation of the skin) in 2 percent of people with the disease. If you think you have "caught" a skin rash from a sexual partner, get to the doctor.

Q *Is it a good idea to "milk" the penis for pus as a follow-up to see if a gonorrhea discharge has stopped?*

A No. You can damage the inner membranes and make the situation worse. Let your doctor do the examining.

Q *Can you get vaginal infections from cunnilingus?*

A Syphilis can be transmitted from the genitals to the

mouth of both sexes, and vice versa. However, evidence for the transmission of other diseases from the mouth to the vagina is slim.

Q *Aren't the breasts sexual organs? Do they get involved in VD?*

A Breasts are called secondary sexual organs and do not have the kind of wet mucous membrane that attracts organisms like syphilis and gonorrhea. However, the thin skin of the nipples is susceptible to scabies mites and physical irritations that may become secondarily infected by nonvenereal bacteria. Syphilis chancres of the breasts have been well documented.

Q *What is the relationship between VD and cancer?*

A This is a bombshell question, of course. There have been some studies that show that women with higher sexual activity, earlier age of onset of sexual activity, and higher pregnancy rate have a higher rate of cancer of the cervix. (The *cervix* is the blind end of the vagina, and the entrance to the womb, or *uterus.*) They also have a higher rate of acquiring venereal disease, but *there is no connection between the two.* It is thought that the more exposure one gets to sexual intercourse, the more exposure one gets to irritants that can cause a breakdown in the normal cells of the cervix that MAY RARELY lead to cancer. Obviously, with more sex with different people, one also runs a higher risk of running into someone with a venereal disease. There is now excellent evidence besides that herpes type 2 virus infection in the female is strongly correlated with cervical cancer. This fits well with other theories about latent viruses as the cause of various types of cancer.

Q *Do men who are uncircumcised run a greater risk of getting a venereal disease than circumcised men?*

A Yes, especially if their hygiene is poor. Women who have intercourse with uncircumcised men have the same vested interest in their hygiene.

Q *Is there anything you can do just after having sex to keep gonorrhea or syphilis germs from "taking" to you, if you have had sex with an infected person?*

A Yes. Believe it or not, simply urinating will clear your passageways and tend to flush out any germs that just got there. This procedure is most effective for men. Showering or taking a bath helps both sexes, and using a bidet tends to remove the offending germs. However, these methods are not foolproof and should not be relied upon exclusively.

Q *What about washing your hands?*

A Cleanliness may or may not be next to godliness, but it is certainly indispensable in its own right. In this age of miracle antibiotics and pills to pop (supposedly) for anything that ails you, people have forgotten the teachings of Lister, Semmelweis, Pasteur, and Schwann about sepsis and antisepsis. Soap and water applied regularly to the hands and body are a great defense against acquiring any kind of infectious disease. Germs, even when they get on or in you from someone else, can frequently be washed away before they get a chance to multiply and cause damage. Even if all the germs present are not washed away, enough will be removed from the battlefield of your body that your natural defenses will be adequate to destroy those that remain.

In other words, wash yourself before and after sex, especially with strangers. A good application of any standard soap with enough water to rinse it off will improve your chances of resisting venereal disease and anything else you might contact by sex (such as colds). Showers are better than baths for men in this respect. For women, showers are more effective for this purpose also, especially since some vaginal foams and jellies require that the woman not take a bath for several hours after sex. If no vaginal foam or jelly has been used, baths, bidets, and/or douches may be taken.

In this age of doing your own thing, some people might say, "I find this insulting and offensive. If you think someone is dirty, why go to bed with him or her in the first place?" Well, no one is in himself "dirty," but germs that may be on him or her are. *No* one is immune to germs, and you don't have to look "dirty" to have a disease. And in the second place you might spot something during or after sex (like a chancre) that you didn't see in the first place.

You don't have to make a great rush for a Clorox bottle the moment you're done; you can approach the subject of washing nonchalantly, simply suggesting a refreshing shower before and/or after sex. A hot shower (alone or with the two of you) can be a delight. Include it in your sexual ritual and you will be doubly rewarded.

Q *Do prostitutes have a high rate of VD?*

A Yes, every form. Twenty percent of prostitutes admitted to prison have gonorrhea. This is 20 times higher than the national average. Prostitutes also have a much higher incidence of syphilis than the rest of the population. There are no safeguards in this country for the legal or paralegal medical inspection of prostitutes as there are in some other countries. Since most prostitutes nowadays work on the street on their own or for a pimp in small groups, there are no longer the elaborate brothels of former years in which a madam could check up on her girls. In other words, the quickness of modern sex works against the health of prostitutes, as it does against everyone else.

Q *Does taking The Pill make you more susceptible to some kinds of VD?*

A Yes! This fact is little known. The Pill contains steroids that are not the ones your body would make normally. Steroids always alter the internal environment and tend to make infection much easier to take hold, and more difficult to eradicate. Women on The Pill have a much higher rate of trichomonal and monilial vaginal infections. These are protozoan and fungal forms, respectively, and the environment of the vagina (acidity, etc.) is changed with The Pill so that they flourish. Millions of women have these irritating vaginal diseases for years without knowing it.

In addition, the risk of acquiring other venereal diseases is probably also increased in women who take The Pill and are exposed to infected men, although there are few studies in the medical literature about this subject.

Q *What about the condom?*

A Our behavior patterns with regard to condoms (elastic rubber prophylactics) provide fascinating insights into our common psyche. In England, people use condoms nonchalantly and regard the use of The Pill as somehow dirty and sordid. In America, The Pill is revered about as highly as the Communion wafer whereas the condom suggests squalid men's rooms in gas stations and dirty people. *As a matter of fact, using the condom is a great help in avoiding venereal disease from an infected partner.* It protects the female from an infected male; it protects the male from an infected female. However, there are severe limitations to its effectiveness. The condom must not have even a minute tear during use or removal, and it must stay on the penis during the entire sexual contact. In no case does it ever cover all the areas susceptible to infection, however; and any kind of oral-genital play, rectal intercourse without the condom, or use of the condom only during the last stages of intercourse will negate its usefulness.

Many people think of the condom only as a device against conception. It is very useful in preventing conception, but cumbersome. With the advent of The Pill, the use of the condom dropped off markedly. Using the condom today therefore seems to imply—to either sex partner—that one fears the other has a venereal disease. We have already established that this is not the subject to bring up in the heat of passion. Therefore, many people find the use of the condom insulting. Nevertheless, if you do not object to using a condom and are having sex with a "dubious" stranger, by all means use one. Condoms could decrease the national epidemic of gonorrhea and other venereal diseases if used in great numbers. *But remember, they are far from foolproof.*

Q *What about "clap" doctors?*

A There are a number of private doctors in big cities who see exclusively patients with gonorrhea and syphilis. Although many of these may be superb physicians, some tend to charge exorbitant fees and do not report their cases to the Public Health Service, which means that the infected contacts of their patients never get help. Although it is wrong to assume that all private physicians who concentrate on a practice of cases of venereal disease are behaving in this way, you should know that there are inexpensive and competent public health clinics in every county of this country where you can get excellent care for your venereal disease problems for little or no money.

Q *What should you do in general to keep on the lookout for VD?*

A The best idea is not to worry about a thing, but to get regular simple checkups. Get an STS blood test for syphilis twice a year at your public health clinic or from a private doctor. If you're a woman, get a vaginal culture for gonorrhea as a routine procedure twice a year from your doctor or from an obstetrics and gynecology clinic. These are the easiest ways to keep a tab on yourself.

Q *What about taking pills like tetracycline or penicillin beforehand to kill off any germs you may come in contact with?*

A If you are an M.D., a bacteriologist, or the like, fine. Otherwise, you are just playing with things that are best left to people who have studied the situation. Inadequate doses of drugs taken before sex will only cause a delay of symptoms and disease. Besides, you can develop allergies to drugs if you take them too often. The best policy in general is don't take any medicine unless you *know* you *have* to.

Q *Are there any occasions when you can treat yourself and not go to the doctor?*

A It is probably unnecessary to go to a doctor for crab lice if nothing else is wrong with you and if you know a crab when you see one. You can buy the insecticide lotions at most drug stores. On the other hand, don't neglect your twice-annual syphilis blood test. And if other symptoms do turn up, go to the doctor and tell him about them.

Q *What about older people who have not checked into their syphilis blood test status? If they have a positive blood test, can they still be helped?*

A Absolutely yes. Everyone should know whether he has a positive or negative syphilis blood test. If the test has been positive for some time, live syphilis spirochetes may still be circulating inside the body, and penicillin can kill them. This is extremely important in averting the late complications of syphilis such as ruptured aorta, mental deterioration, and so on. It is never too late to check one's blood test for syphilis and to try a course of penicillin. The real tragedy of the Tuskegee study of the 1930s and 1940s was that once penicillin was discovered, it was not given to the patients who had tested the older treatments of heavy metals and other methods. Even in cases where the syphilis germs have done irreversible anatomical damage to the blood vessels, it is helpful to the physician to know the origin of the damage, which he may not attribute to syphilis otherwise.

Q *Can blood tests for syphilis be reversed? That is, if you get a positive blood test, can giving penicillin change it to negative?*

A YES, up to a point. If the patient has a positive blood test, that means he has had syphilis at some point and may not have been treated or has received treatment too late or too little. After many years of a positive blood test it is impossible to revert the test to negative, but the strength of the positive reaction can be diluted and live syphilis organisms in the body can be killed with large doses of antibiotics.

If the patient has had a positive blood test for only a few weeks or months, the test usually reverts to negative altogether with proper treatment. It is necessary to have repeat blood tests to follow the decrease of the positive reaction to zero to have complete assurance that the disease has indeed been cured.

Q *What is the prospect for the VD epidemic rate at the present time?*

A Up, up, and away, unless people understand what they are facing—infectious diseases that can be quickly treated with medical care—and unless those who are sexually active get regular checkups and see that their sexual contacts are treated when a venereal problem does turn up.

Chapter Ten:

WHERE DO YOU GO FOR HELP?

Where should people go for help with venereal diseases? The answer depends on where you live, how you get your medical care, and whom you choose to see. Many family doctors have learned to deal with the problems of gonorrhea, syphilis, and so on with great expertise. If you feel that your doctor is old-fashioned or maybe a little behind the times and you do not wish to go to him, find another one. Call your local public health service and ask them to recommend a VD clinic. In small communities or rural areas, there is usually a county health department in every county seat, with branches in other communities. They may have a separate VD clinic or may see you in a general clinic. Every state capital has a state bureau of health that is responsible for looking after the medical health of the state as a whole; if you call your state government general operator or the state bureau of health, someone will direct you to a public VD clinic in your area.

In large urban areas, most city governments have city public health clinics, with separate VD clinic divisions. You can call your local city health department and ask them where to go.

In recent years, starting on the West Coast, some free "street clinics" have developed, particularly in San Francisco, Oakland, Berkeley, and Los Angeles, which provide free VD diagnosis and treatment. These clinics regrettably often perform their diagnosis and treatment without asking about your contacts. Some doctors—particularly public health doctors—find this lack of follow-up negligent; but such treatment is better than nothing.

In the past couple of years an organization has been founded in Philadelphia called Operation Venus. The organizer was a then high-school senior named Joseph J. Forish, who is now only a college junior. The group is well organized and is run by teen-agers for teen-agers, although if you are no longer a teen-ager they will be glad to help you anyway. You may call *toll-free* from anywhere in the country, including Alaska and Hawaii, to the national headquarters by dialing 800-523-1885 between the hours of 9 A.M. and 9 P.M. eastern standard (or daylight) time. There are trained people who man the phones and can discuss particular symptoms and treatment with you. They can suggest doctors and clinics in your own community where you can go and often indicate where treatment can be gotten *free.* You don't have to give your name unless you want written material sent to you. The opportunity to talk to someone of your own age group who understands and can point you in the right direction is a great help in facing the problem of venereal diseases.

In addition, there are local Operation Venus hotlines in communities around the country that may be dialed free within the state.

For Philadelphia locally, dial 215-567-6969.

For Pennsylvania (outside Philadelphia), dial 215-567-6973. Some of the local branches of the groups cooperating with the national Operation Venus program have had their phone numbers changed; so rather than print a lot of obsolete numbers here, we suggest you call the national number or use your local telephone directory to obtain the numbers of community VD clinics.

If you are still at a loss after exhausting these means, call the nearest hospital and ask the information operator or a doctor on call in the emergency room where you may receive help. If you wish to be helped, you can get help.

The fee in public health clinics is little or nothing. Blood tests for syphilis are provided free on demand in some cases, whether or not you have a symptom of the disease or not. Medical personnel are only too eager to help with these problems in the light of the current epidemic.

Q *What about public health caseworkers. Don't they blab?*

A Public health personnel are neither police nor judges, and they lose their jobs automatically if they break the confidence of the people they are helping. Some work for the United States Public Health Service and are responsible to the Center for Disease Control in Atlanta, Georgia. Others are paid by city and state governments. They are trained medical and sociological professionals, with a deep loyalty to your health needs. They have seen too much of life and of disease to be shocked or titillated by anything you have to tell them and are interested only in getting people to treatment and then going on to the next case. They do not record your health status on your permanent work record or with the police, the FBI, or any other arm of the law, real or imagined. Information about you is kept confidential and is not given even to other doctors in your community unless you request it. Even superiors in the public health service cannot look at the records unless a valid reason is presented and kept on permanent file. There is no idle gossip over coffee and Danish. You will not walk down Main Street branded for life, nor should you feel any stigma attached to helping one of your sexual partners get medical care.

Chapter Eleven:

SEX AND THE SIMPLE WORD: An Eclectic Glossary of Venereal Disease

QUESTION: Why do doctors use such fancy words for diseases and parts of the anatomy? ANSWER: Every line of work has its own particular jargon. In the case of medicine, where millions of facts must be systematized to be remembered or retrieved easily, conventional prefixes, root words, and suffixes have developed over the centuries. Because all scientific learning was for hundreds of years transmitted through the exacting medium of the Latin language, many Latin naming systems have survived and are still very useful. Names that may seem obscure or even deliberately difficult to you have a rationale that, once mastered, provides an easy source of understanding for similar words in the future.

In the case of the venereal diseases, because of the sexual charge of the problems we are discussing, there are often commonly used nicknames for parts of the anatomy and illnesses in question. This glossary attempts to list all the "correct" names in alphabetical order and explain them, with popular synonyms given where they are applicable.

anus (A-nus), n. The external outlet of the rectum; the skin around the outlet of the lower intestine; asshole.

asymptomatic, adj. Nonsymptomatic. That is, not giving any indication of a particular disease. People who have a disease and do not feel anything from it are said to be asymptomatic.

"blood test," n. A much abused and meaningless term circulated by the general public, generally with knowing nods. There are many kinds of "blood tests" for many different medical problems. The term should be abandoned. See **VDRL** and **Wassermann.**

Candida albicans, n. The formal name for the species of yeast that causes thrush, an inflammation of the mouth, or vaginal irritation. The organism is also called *monilia*. The disease caused by the spread of this fungus therefore is called either *moniliasis* or *candidiasis*.

canker (KANG-ker), n. A general descriptive term for any kind of eroding ulcer, usually in reference to one in the mouth, from any cause, as from irritating chemicals, viruses, etc.

cervix (SER-viks), n. From the Latin, literally meaning "neck." As applied to the reproductive anatomy, it means the neck of the womb **(uterus)**, which connects the womb to the end of the vagina. The cervix has a small opening through which sperm travel from the vagina through the womb. The cervix is not to be confused with the hymen, a thin, temporary membrane at the front or head of the vagina. The cervix is a strong and sturdy structure. With regard to venereal diseases, the cervix is often the site of monilial and trichomonal infection, and in cases of gonorrhea, pus frequently gathers near the cervix.

chancre (SHANG-ker), n. From the French. Now used to mean specifically the sore or lesion of primary syphilis, a raised, generally painless ulcer usually on the male and female genitals, but sometimes occurring on the tongue or other parts of the body. A chancre is highly infectious to other people and is teeming with syphilis germs (spirochetes).

chancroid (SHANG-kroid), n. Literally means "resembling a chancre." Also called *soft chancre.* Refers specifically to the sore or lesion or ulcer of *chancroid disease,* and *not* of syphilis. The chancroid sore is usually painful and indicates a local infection by the Ducrey bacillus as opposed to the syphilis germ, which causes damage throughout the body. Syphilis is much more dangerous, but only a doctor who does the right tests can be sure he can tell the difference.

clap, n. Usually referred to as "the clap." A slang expression for all forms of gonorrhea, also called GC, the dose.

clitoris, n. A small midline erectile organ in the female where the *labia minora* (smaller folds) of the vulva come together. This organ is homologous to the penis in the male. It is rarely affected by venereal disease.

condom, n. An elastic rubber balloon that fits over the penis that, when properly used, prevents transmission of sperm or germs from the male to the female, and of germs from the female to the male. Only one kind of many "prophylactics." Commonly called a rubber.

condyloma (kon-di-LO-mah), n. A general term for a wart. Plural is *condylomata.* Usually used in reference to anal, genital, or perineal warts. *Condylomata lata* ("broad warts") refer specifically to the highly infectious warts of syphilis. *Condylomata acuminata* are warts due to relatively innocent viruses and have nothing to do with syphilis, although they can be annoying and are spreadable from one person to the next.

conjunctivitis (kon-junk-te-VI-tis), n. An inflammation of the whites of the eyes, from any cause. Gonorrhea can cause conjunctivitis in newborn babies delivered of infected mothers; the conjunctivitis in these infants can progress quickly to complete blindness.

crabs, n. A nickname for the disease of pediculosis, or infestation by "crab" lice *(Phthirus pubis)*. Also used to refer to the lice themselves.

cunnilingus, n. Oral contact with the female genitals. From the Latin.

cystitis, n. Inflammation of the bladder, which is structurally a "cyst." Infection of the female bladder can occur as a consequence of trauma (any kind of damage, as by abrasion) after the first sexual intercourse. In that case, "honeymoon cystitis" is spoken of.

discharge, n. Any kind of drip, normal or abnormal, from any opening in the body. Many of the diseases in this book are first noticed because of their discharges.

epididymis (Ep-e-DID-e-mis), n. The mass of tubes and tissues that spiral out from the substance of each testicle. Through the epididymis the testicle is connected to the rest of the male genitourinary tract. Sperm cells originate in the testicular tissue and pass to the urethra through the epididymis.

fellatio, n. Mouth contact of any kind with the penis. A not uncommon heterosexual and homosexual practice. Recently pinpointed in the medical literature as a transmission point of such venereal diseases as gonorrhea.

genitals, n., always plural. From the Latin, meaning things that beget. Refers to male and/or female sexual organs, exterior and/or interior. Breasts are secondary sexual characteristics and are *not* genitals.

genitourinary tract. In both men and women, the systems that produce and eliminate urine and that produce and transmit and develop sperm and egg cells originate from the same primitive cell mass. Thus reproductive and urinary systems are anatomically and embryologically interrelated and often are involved in disease processes together. For these reasons the reproductive and the urinary systems are frequently referred to together as the genitourinary tract.

"gonococcus," n. An accepted slang term used widely in medical and nonmedical circles to indicate the organism that causes gonorrhea, which organism is correctly termed *Neisseria gonorrhoeae*. A small bacterium.

gonorrhea, n. From the Latin, meaning discharge in the sexual organs. A disease caused by the specific bacterial species, *Neisseria gonorrhoeae*, affecting the sexual organs by local invasion and, infrequently, spreading through the blood to distant organs. Commonly called the clap, the dose, GC.

granuloma inguinale, n. Latin descriptive name for a disease, meaning "inguinal diseased scar formation." A specific disease involving local invasion and destruction of the groin tissue and caused by the bacteria formerly called *Donovania granulomatis* and just recently reclassified as *Calymmatobacterium granulomatis*.

groin, n. Technically, the fold between the lower abdomen and the thigh. Generally it means the entire region of the lower abdomen, the genitals, and the upper thigh.

hemorrhoids, n. Abnormal swollen veins in the rectum, distended and usually painful to one degree or another. May be irritated and secondarily infected by rectal intercourse. Have nothing to do themselves with venereal disease.

hepatitis, n. A general term meaning inflammation of the liver, from any cause. Generally used to refer to "infectious hepatitis" or "serum hepatitis," two variations on a serious liver infection by the same elusive specific virus. The virus of hepatitis lives not only in the liver but also in the intestinal tract and may be picked up by another person engaged in oral-anal, oral-perineal, or even oral-genital contact with a person in the infectious stages of hepatitis. One symptom of hepatitis is jaundice, or yellowness. "Jaundice" is *not* synonymous with "hepatitis."

herpes simplex, n. The technical name for the species of virus of which several types cause fever blisters on the mouth and very painful similar ulcers on the sexual organs. A common venereal disease is *herpes genitalis,* or herpes of the sexual organs.

hymen, n. The thin membrane at the entrance to the vagina. The narrow passage in it present at birth is widened to afford entrance of the penis. Spoken of as the "cherry" in common slang.

incubation period. The time between actual entry of a germ onto or into your body and the time that symptoms start developing from the germs as they multiply. In a sense, a "latent" period, although not the long "latent" period of syphilis.

infect, v. To invade and significantly alter the internal functioning of an organism. Generally, bacteria and viruses are said to "infect" a person because they cause many internal changes and may even destroy essential internal tissues.

infest, v. To live off, or parasitize, an organism. Lice are said to infest persons because they stay on the surface and do not corrupt the internal integrity of the organism being parasitized.

—itis, suffix. A common ending for many medical words, it means inflammation or irritation, whether from an infectious or a purely mechanical source.

jaundice, n. From the French: yellowness. A simple physical descriptive term, it may indicate hepatitis or any number of other causes.

labia majora, n., plural. Latin, literally "big lips." The outer two symmetrical folds of the vulva that frame the opening to the vagina.

labia minora, n., plural. Latin, literally "smaller lips." The inner two symmetrical folds of the vulva that frame the opening to the vagina. The clitoris is found between the two labia minora at their junction atop the opening.

latent period. Medically, any portion of the evolution of a disease in which nothing seems wrong with the patient while disease processes continue internally to subvert the normal function of the individual. In syphilis, the latent period often occurs after symptoms have died down and lasts for years before major complications finally show up.

lesion, n. A nonspecific term referring to the unit of injury; a pockmark is *the* lesion of smallpox; a chancre is *a* lesion of syphilis. A wound; a hurt.

leukorrhea (LU-ko-RE-ah), n. From the Greek, meaning a discharge of white material. Hence, any abnormal discharge in which broken-down white blood cells are present; the white color of the discharge indicates a white blood cell response to an irritation or infection. Pus is massive leukorrhea.

louse, n. Literally, a tiny parasitic insect. Plural is *lice,* adjectival form is *lousy.* All figurative usages derive from these meanings.

lymph node, n. Part of the body's system of immune defense against infection. The lymphatic system is separate from the blood vessels and has its own vessels that often run parallel to blood vessels. Lymph nodes occur at intervals along the lymphatic vessels and serve (1) to produce lymph cells that attack bacteria and produce antibodies and (2) to filter germs that come in through the skin. When germs are present in large numbers, the nodes may be overwhelmed, swell up, drain pus, and feel extremely painful. Thus swollen lymph nodes are a sign of a particularly difficult challenge to the body's defenses from some invader in the area of the node.

lymphogranuloma venereum, n. A disease caused by a *Chlamydia* organism and affecting the lymph glands of the groin and perineum. Confused sometimes with syphilis, chancroid, and granuloma inguinale.

monilia, n. plural. See *Candida albicans.*

mononucleosis, n. A disease of the lymph nodes characterized by a proliferation of a certain type of blood cell (the "mononuclear" cell) and caused by a specific virus. The disease may mimic the symptoms of infectious hepatitis.

nit, n. A louse egg.

nonspecific urethritis. A general condition of irritation of the urethra (see below) that is often mistaken for gonorrhea and in fact can be distinguished from gonorrhea only by painstaking culture methods. Nonspecific urethritis is also called nongonococcal urethritis. It is a recurrent condition and hard to eradicate and can be communicated sexually from one person to the next.

ovary, n. The egg-producing female sexual organ, linked to the womb by the oviducts.

oviduct, n. From the Latin, literally "egg leading." The organ that physically links the ovaries and the womb and transports the eggs from the ovaries to the womb. Synonym: Fallopian tube.

pediculosis, n. The state of being infested with crab lice.

pelvis, n. The bones and contents of the inner lower abdomen. The sexual organs of the female are all contained within the pelvis.

penis, n. The male organ of erectile tissue. The outlet at the end of the penis is the outlet of the urethra, the tube that carries urine from the bladder to the outside and semen from the male sexual glands to the outside. Commonly called prick, etc. Adjectival form is *penile*.

perineum (PER-i-NE-um) n. Generally, the base or outlet of the pelvis. The perineum includes the external sexual organs, the anus, and the skin surface between them.

Phthirus pubis, n. The official name for crab lice.

PID (pelvic inflammatory disease). The condition in which gonorrhea in the female progresses to the point of spreading pus throughout the oviducts and over the ovaries, obstructing the natural spaces of the oviducts and frequently causing peritonitis and sterility.

prepuce, (PRE-pus), n. The foreskin of the penis.

prophylactic, n. or adj. Literally, anything that guards against or stands in the way of disease. Often used to refer specifically to a condom, or rubber.

prostate, n. An inflexible internal organ of the male sexual system in which the tube of the urethra begins. Not to be confused with "prostrate," which means laid out flat on the floor.

pruritus (proo-RI-tus), n. Itching.

rectum, n. The last part of the lower intestine or colon. The rectum is an internal organ; its external outlet is called the anus.

scabies (SKA-beez), n. "The itch," mange; the state of infestation with the mite called *Sarcoptes scabiei,* the human agent of mange.

symptom (SIMP-tum), n. Any noticeable change of the

body's appearance or function indicating a disease. Adjectival form is *symptomatic.*

syphilis (SIF-i-lis), n. Synonym: lues. A systemic infection by the spirochete germ *Treponema pallidum,* first affecting the sexual organs, where it generally but not exclusively gains entry to the body, and then spreading by the blood to all the organs of the body. The syphilis spirochete germ can live for decades in the body, slowly causing destruction of many different tissues and body functions. Over the centuries, few diseases have caused as much misery as syphilis. Now easily treated by penicillin and other antibiotics.

tabes dorsalis (TA-beeze dor-SA-lis), n. A complication of syphilis affecting a certain part of the spinal cord nervous function and manifesting itself in a characteristic peculiar gait of the sufferer. Irreversible once it has developed.

testicle, n. The primary male sexual gland; the ball containing the *testis,* where sperm are manufactured. Spoken of in pairs, as *testicles.* Synonyms: balls, nuts, etc.

Treponema pallidum (trep-o-NE-mah PAL-e-dum), n. The official name for the bacterium that, in the plural, causes syphilis. A particular type of *spirochete,* an order of bacteria characterized by a long, slender, corkscrew-like shape.

Trichomonas vaginalis (TRI-kom-o-nas VAJ-i-NAH-lis), n. A particular Protozoa that causes the itch and discharge of *trichomoniasis.* Can affect both sexes, but causes more symptoms in the female. The organism is also called a *trichomonad.*

ureter (U-re-ter), n. The tube that connects and delivers urine from the kidney to the bladder. There are two ureters in the normal person, one from each kidney to the (same) bladder.

urethra (u-RE-thrah), n. The tube that connects the bladder with the outside. Men and women both have urethras; the male urethra ends at the tip of the penis and the female urethra, which is much shorter, ends at the vaginal outlet.

uterus (U-ter-us), n. The womb; the muscular organ in

which sperm cells meet egg cells normally, are implanted on the surface, and develop into a fetus.

vagina (vah-JI-nah), n. Latin, meaning literally a sheath or scabbard. The canal that leads from the external female sexual outlet to the cervix and womb. A "sheath" for the penis. There is no single word that refers specifically and exclusively to the vagina, but it is commonly called the "birth canal."

vaginitis, n. The state of itching in the vagina, from whatever cause.

VDRL. An acronym for Venereal Diseases Research Laboratory, the laboratory of the Center for Disease Control in Atlanta; the term is commonly used to mean the specific "blood test" for syphilis developed by that laboratory as an improvement on the classic Wassermann test.

venereal, adj. From the Latin, Venus, Veneris, third-declension feminine noun, the goddess of love. Venery means lovemaking; venereal means anything to do with lovemaking and usually refers specifically to sexual intercourse.

vulva (VUL-vah), n. All the external parts of the female sexual organs; that is, the labia majora and minora, the clitoris, and the hymen.

Wassermann. An obsolete term referring to the test developed over 60 years ago by August von Wassermann, a German pioneer bacteriologist, which indicates the presence of syphilis in the body.

APPENDIX A*

Recommended Treatment Schedules for Gonorrhea

March 1972

For *Neisseria gonorrhoeae* infection the preferred drug is penicillin G or ampicillin. Physicians are cautioned to use no less than the recommended doses of antibiotics.

For Treatment of Uncomplicated Gonorrhea (Urethral, Cervical, Pharyngeal, or Rectal)

Parenteral—Men or Women—Aqueous procaine penicillin G, 4.8 million units intramuscularly divided into at least two doses and injected at different sites at one visit, together with 1 gram of oral probenecid, preferably given at least 30 minutes prior to the injection.

OR

Oral—Men or Women—Ampicillin, 3.5 grams, with probenecid, 1 gram, administered simultaneously.

Treatment of contacts: Patients with known exposure to gonorrhea should receive the same treatment as those known to have gonorrhea.

*U. S. Department of Health, Education, and Welfare, Public Health Service, Health Services & Mental Health Administration, Center for Disease Control, State and Community Services Division, Venereal Disease Branch, Atlanta, Georgia 30333.

When Penicillin or Ampicillin is Contraindicated,* or When the Above Schedules Are Ineffective

Parenteral—Men—Spectinomycin, 2 grams, in one intramuscular injection.
Women—Spectinomycin, 4 grams, in one intramuscular injection.

OR

Oral—Men or Women—Tetracycline HCl, 1.5 grams initially, followed by 0.5 gram four times a day for 4 days, a total dosage of 9 grams. Other tetracyclines are not more effective.

Follow-Up

It is desirable that follow-up urethral cultures be obtained from males 7 days after completion of treatment; it is desirable that cervical and rectal cultures be obtained from females 7–14 days after completion of treatment.

Complications

Although treatment of complications (gonococcal salpingitis, bacteremia, arthritis, etc.) must be individualized, repeated large parenteral doses of aqueous crystalline penicillin G have been shown to be effective. The efficacy of alternative antibiotic regimens is unproven. Postgonococcal urethritis can be treated with tetracycline, 0.5 gram, orally four times a day for at least 7 days.

*Allergy to penicillin, ampicillin, probenecid, or previous anaphylactic reaction.

Syphilis

All gonorrhea patients should have a serologic test for syphilis at the time of diagnosis. Patients receiving the recommended parenteral penicillin schedule need not have follow-up serologic tests for syphilis. Patients treated with ampicillin, spectinomycin, or tetracycline should have a follow-up serologic test for syphilis each month for 4 months to detect syphilis that may have been masked by treatment for gonorrhea.

Patients with gonorrhea who also have syphilis should be given additional treatment appropriate to the stage of syphilis.

While long-acting forms of penicillin (such as benzathine penicillin G) are effective in syphilotherapy, they have *NO* place in the treatment of gonorrhea.

APPENDIX B*

Recommended Treatment Schedules for Syphilis

Primary, Secondary Syphilis

Rx: Benzathine penicillin G—2.4 million units total (1.2 million units in each buttock) by intramuscular injection.

OR:

PAM—4.8 million units total usually given 2.4 million units at first session, as above, and 1.2 million units at each of two subsequent injections 3 days apart.

OR:

Aqueous procaine penicillin G—600,000 units daily for 8 days to total 4.8 million units.

Latent Syphilis

Rx: Benzathine penicillin G—If no spinal fluid examination is done, treatment must encompass the possibility of asymptomatic neurosyphilis. In this case, 6.0-9.0 million units total, given 3.0 million units (1.5 in each buttock each session) at 7-day interval.

*U. S. Department of Health, Education, and Welfare, Public Health Service, Health Services & Mental Health Administration, Center for Disease Control, State and Community Services Division, Venereal Disease Branch, Atlanta, Georgia 30333.

With nonreactive spinal fluid examination, 2.4 million units (as primary).

OR:

PAM—Aqueous penicillin G—Same as primary syphilis.

Congenital Syphilis

Rx: Benzathine penicillin G—50,000 units per kilogram of body weight at one clinic visit.*

OR:

Aqueous Procaine Penicillin G—100,000 units per kilogram of body weight divided into daily dosage over 10-day period.*

Late Syphilis

Asymptomatic neurosyphilis
Symptomatic neurosyphilis
Cardiovascular syphilis
Late benign (cutaneous, osseous, and visceral gumma) syphilis
Rx: Benzathine penicillin G—6.0 to 9.0 million units total, given 3.0 million units at 7-day intervals.

OR:

PAM—6.0-9.0 million units total, given 1.2 million units at 3-day intervals.

OR:

Aqueous procaine penicillin G—6.0 to 9.0 million units total, given 600,000 units daily.
Any benefit from more than 10 million units has not been demonstrated.

Syphilis in Pregnancy

Syphilis in pregnancy should be managed in the same

*Total dosage not to exceed 5.0-6.0 million units.

manner as with any non-pregnant patient. Urgency of treatment is the keynote to therapy.

Alternate Antibiotics

When sensitivity precludes use of penicillin, erythromycin and tetracycline are the best alternate drugs. Recommended dosage orally is 30-40 gms. of erythromycin and 30-40 gms. of tetracycline given over a period of 10–15 days.

Treatment with such alternate antibiotics must be accompanied by close follow-up of the syphilitic patient since none of these drugs has had adequate evaluation in all stages of syphilis. Spinal fluid examinations must be done as part of follow-up after this type of therapy.

Preventive Treatment

If the patient is known to have been exposed to lesion syphilis, it is a fallacy to wait for the disease to develop to the clinical or reactive serologic stage, meanwhile allowing reinfection of treated patients and the infection of additional persons. However, every effort should be made to arrive at a diagnosis, including a complete physical examination, before administering preventive treatment.

Adequate preventive treatment may consist of 2.4 million units of benzathine penicillin G.

BIBLIOGRAPHY

Nearly all of the works consulted below are intended for readers able to understand technical medical terms. Nevertheless, the general texts may provide interesting reading in depth for someone who has been stimulated by the present volume.

Books

U.S. Department of Health, Education, and Welfare, Public Health Service. *Syphilis: A Synopsis*. Washington, D.C.: U.S. Government Printing Office, Public Health Service Publication No. 1660, January, 1968.

Brown, William J., Donohue, James F., Axnick, Norman W., Blount, Joseph H., Ewen, Neal H., and Jones, Oscar G. *Syphilis and Other Venereal Diseases*. American Public Health Association Vital and Health Statistics Monographs. Cambridge, Mass.: Harvard University Press, 1970.

King, Ambrose, and Nicol, Claude. *Venereal Diseases,* 2d ed. Philadelphia: F. A. Davis Company, 1969.

Faust, Ernest Carroll, Russell, Paul Farr, and Jung, Rodney Clifton. *Craig and Faust's Clinical Parasitology,* 8th rev. ed. Philadelphia: Lea & Febiger, 1970.

Beeson, Paul B., and McDermott, Walsh, eds. *Cecil-Loeb Textbook of Medicine,* 12th rev. ed. Philadelphia: W. B. Saunders Company, 1967.

Schwartz, Seymour I., editor-in-chief. *Principles of Surgery*. New York: McGraw-Hill Book Company, Blakiston Division, 1969.

Dubos, Rene J., and Hirsch, James G., eds. *Bacterial and Mycotic Infections of Man,* 4th rev. ed. Philadelphia: J. B. Lippincott Company, 1965.

Grimble, A. S. *McLachlan's Handbook of Diagnosis and Treatment of Venereal Diseases,* 5th rev. ed. London: E. and S. Livingstone Ltd., 1969.

Webster, Bruce, guest editor. Symposium on Venereal Diseases. *Medical Clinics of North America,* vol. 56, no. 5. Philadelphia: W. B. Saunders Company, September, 1972.

U.S. Department of Health, Education, and Welfare, Public Health Service. Center for Disease Control, Venereal Disease Branch. *Management of Chancroid, Granuloma Inguinale, Lymphogranuloma Venereum in General Practice.* Washington: Public Health Service Publication No. 255, rev. ed. 1964.

Meaker, Samuel Raynor. *A Doctor Talks to Women: What They Should Know About the Normal Functions and Common Disorders of the Female Organs.* New York: Simon and Schuster, 1954.

The Diagnosis of Gonorrhea: A Programmed Physician Review. New York: Pfizer Laboratories, 1971.

The Treatment of Gonorrhea: A Programmed Review for Physicians. New York: Pfizer Laboratories, 1971.

Rosebury, Theodor. *Microbes and Morals: The Strange Story of Venereal Disease.* New York: The Viking Press, 1971.

Nesselrod, J. Peerman. *Clinical Proctology,* 3d rev. ed. Philadelphia: W. B. Saunders Company, 1964.

Turrell, Robert, ed. *Diseases of the Colon and Anorectum,* 2d rev. ed. Philadelphia: W. B. Saunders Company, 1969.

Journals

Clark, Matthew. "VD: The Epidemic." *Newsweek,* January 24, 1972, pp. 46-50.

U.S. Department of Health, Education, and Welfare, Public Health Service, Health Services and Mental Health Administration, Center for Disease Control. *Current Literature on Venereal Disease.* Atlanta: Venereal Disease Branch. Published three or four times annually.

The VD Crisis, from the proceedings of the International Venereal Disease Symposium, St. Louis, Missouri, 1971. New York: Pfizer Laboratories Division, 1971.

Today's VD Control Problem. New York: American Social Health Association, 1972.

Darrow, William W. *Selected References on the Behavioral Aspects of Venereal Disease Control: An Annotated Bibliography for Behavioral Scientists, Epidemiologists, and Venereal Disease Casefinding Personnel.* U.S. Department of Health, Education, and Welfare, Public Health Service. Atlanta: Health Services and Mental Health Administration, Center for Disease Control.

U.S. Department of Health, Education, and Welfare, Public Health Service, Health Services and Mental Health Administration, *The Laboratory Aspects of Syphilis.* Atlanta: Center for Disease Control, Venereal Disease Branch, May, 1971.

U.S. Department of Health, Education, and Welfare, Public Health Service, Health Services and Mental Health Administration. *Principal Recommendations of the National Commission on Venereal Disease.* Atlanta: Center for Disease Control, Venereal Disease Branch, 1971.

U.S. Department of Health, Education, and Welfare, Public Health Service, Health Services and Mental Health Administration. *Morbidity and Mortality.* Atlanta: Center for Disease Control, a weekly report on the infectious diseases.

U.S. Department of Health, Education, and Welfare, Public Health Service, Health Services and Mental Health Administration. *VD Fact Sheet 1971: Basic Statistics on the Venereal Disease Problem in the United States.* Atlanta: Center for Disease Control, Venereal Disease Branch, DHEW Publication no. (HSM) 72-8085, 1971.

Holmes, King K., Johnson, David W., and Trostle, Henry J. "An Estimate of the Risk of Men Acquiring Gonorrhea by Sexual Contact with Infected Females." *American Journal of Epidemiology,* vol. 91, no. 2, 1970.

Nazarian, Lawrence F. "Gonorrhea in Children." *Medical Aspects of Human Sexuality,* May, 1972, pp. 50-61.

Fiumara, Nicholas J., Wise, Henry M., Jr., and Many, Moshe. "Gonorrheal Pharyngitis." *New England Journal of Medicine 276*:1248-1250 (June 1), 1967.

Dunlop, E. M. C., Jones, Barrie R., Darougar, S., and Treharne, J. D. "Chlamydia and Non-specific Urethritis." *British Medical Journal 2*:575-577 (3 June), 1972.

Schroeter, Arnold L., and Pazin, George J. "Gonorrhea." *Annals of Internal Medicine 72*:553-559, April, 1970. Available from the U.S. Department of Health, Education, and Welfare, Public Health Service, CDC, Atlanta, Georgia.

Lucas, James B. "Gonococcal Resistance to Antibiotics." *Southern Medical Bulletin 59*:22-28, April, 1971.

Ackerman, A. Bernard. "Crabs—The Resurgence of *Phthirus pubis*." *New England Journal of Medicine 278*: 950-951 (April 25), 1968.

Fleming, William L., Brown, William J., Donohue, James F., and Branigin, Paul W. "National Survey of Venereal Disease Treated by Physicians in 1968." *Journal of the American Medical Association 211*:1827-1830 (March 16), 1970.

"Venereal Disease Remains Major Health Problem." *Journal of the American Medical Association 221*:14-15 (July 3), 1972.

Altchek, Albert. "Epidemic Pediculosis and Gonorrhea." *Obstetrics and Gynecology 35*:638-641 (April), 1970.

Alexander, J. O'D. "Scabies and Pediculosis." *The Practitioner 200*:632-644 (May), 1968.

Wilkinson, A. E. "Serology of Syphilis." *British Medical Journal*, 573-575 (3 June), 1972.

Dunn, Frederick L. "Fur, Lice, and History." A Letter in *Science 154*:846-847 (18 November), 1966.

Cornelius, Chalmers M. "Rising Gonorrhea a Threat to Vision." U.S. Department of Health, Education, and Welfare, Public Health Service, CDC Publication, Atlanta, Georgia.

Thatcher, Richard W., McCraney, Ward T., Kellogg, Douglas S., and Whaley, William H. "Asymptomatic Gonorrhea." *Journal of the American Medical Association 210*:315-317 (October 13), 1969. Available from the U.S. Department of Health, Education, and Welfare, Public Health Service, CDC, Atlanta.

Owen, Robert L., and Hill, J. Lawrence. "Rectal and Pharyngeal Gonorrhea in Homosexual Men." *Journal of the American Medical Association 220*:1315-1318 (June 5), 1972.

Holmes, King K., Counts, George W., and Beaty, Harry N. "Disseminated Gonococcal Infection." *Annals of Internal Medicine 74*:979-993 (June), 1971.

Pariser, Harry, and Marino, A. F. "Gonorrhea—Frequently Unrecognized Reservoirs." *Southern Medical Journal 63*: 198-201 (February), 1970.

"Lymphogranuloma Venereum." *Medical Aspects of Human Sexuality,* 132-138 (January), 1972.

Arnold, Charles B., and Cogswell, Betty E. "A Condom Distribution Program for Adolescents: The Findings of a Feasibility Study." *American Journal of Public Health 61*: 739-750 (April), 1971.

Kilpatrick, Zachary M. "Gonorrheal Proctitis." *New England Journal of Medicine 287*:967-969 (November 9), 1972.

McCormack, William M., Braun, Peter, Lee, Yhu-Hsiung, Klein, Jerome O., and Kass, Edward H. "The Genital Mycoplasmas." *New England Journal of Medicine 288*:77-89 (January 11), 1973.

Halverstadt, Donald B. "Venereal Warts." *Medical Aspects of Human Sexuality,* 12-21 (June), 1972.

Israel, S. Leon. "The Vaginal Douche: A Gynecologic Anachronism." *Obstetrics and Gynecology 1*:591-592 (May), 1953.

Glynn, Robert. "Daily Douching: Effect on Vaginal Mucosa." *Obstetrics and Gynecology 22*:640-642 (November), 1963.

Egenolf, George F., and McNaughton, Robert H. F. "Chemical Peritonitis Resulting from Vaginal Douche." *Obstetrics and Gynecology 7*:23-24 (January), 1956.

Barnes, Josephine. "Uses and Abuses of Vaginal Douching." *The Practitioner 184*:668-670 (January), 1960.

Glynn, Robert. "Vaginal pH and the Effect of Douching." *Obstetrics and Gynecology 20*:369-372 (September), 1962.

Hirst, Donald V. "Dangers of Improper Vaginal Douching." *American Journal of Obstetrics and Gynecology 64*: 179-183 (July), 1952.

McGowan, Larry. "Peritonitis Following the Vaginal Douche and a Proposed Alternative Method for Vaginal and Vulvar Care." *American Journal of Obstetrics and Gynecology 93*:506-509 (October 15), 1965.

Dodge, Eva F. "The Doctor Talks about Feminine Hygiene." *Journal of the American Medical Women's Association 27*:146-154 (March), 1972.

Wiesner, Paul J., Tronca, Evelyn, Bonin, Paul, Pedersen, Alf H. B., and Holmes, King K. "Clinical Spectrum of Pharyngeal Gonococcal Infection." *New England Journal of Medicine 288*:181-185 (January 25), 1973.

"The 40-Year Death Watch." *Medical World News,* 15-17 (August 18), 1972.

Sparling, P. Frederick. "Medical Progress: Diagnosis and Treatment of Syphilis." *New England Journal of Medicine 284*:642-653 (March 25), 1971.

Swett, Carlton E. "Pilonidal Cyst." *The Journal of the Maine Medical Association,* 272-273 (November), 1971.

Campbell, Edward D. "Changing Concepts in the Treatment of Pilonidal Disease." *The American Journal of Proctology 20*:206-208 (June), 1969.

Gallagher, John Q. "Sacrococcygeal Pilonidal Disease." *Surgical Clinics of North America 49*:1223-1226 (December), 1969.

Zimmerman, Karl. "Pilonidal Disease." *Diseases of the Colon and Rectum 13*:330-332 (July-August), 1970.

Stephens, F. O., and Sloane, D. R. "Conservative Management of Pilonidal Sinus." *Surgery, Gynecology & Obstetrics 129*:786-788 (October), 1969.

Thomas, David. "Pilonidal Sinus: A Review of the Literature and a Report of 100 Cases." *The Medical Journal of Australia,* 184-188 (July 27), 1968.

Darrow, William W. "Is the V.D. Patient Really Sick? A Sociological Analysis of Syphilis, Gonorrhea and the Sick Role in Contemporary American Society." Presented at the American Public Health Association Section on Epidemiology and Behavioral Aspects of Venereal Disease Control, Minneapolis, Minnesota, October 14, 1971. Mimeographed, 8 pages.

INDEX

ABOUT THE AUTHOR

DR. JOHN J. SECONDI, received his M.D. from the Vanderbilt University School of Medicine in Nashville, Tennessee, and is now a New York State licensed practitioner. The results of his independent research have been published in the AMERICAN JOURNAL OF CLINICAL NUTRITION and he writes a column for FAMILY WEEKLY MAGAZINE. He has produced documentary films and edited accompanying monographs on wound healing, gout, peptic ulcer diseases and anxiety. Dr. Secondi has also been the consultant for many medical films and, recently, both author and consultant for eight videotape shows on gastrointestinal disease for the Network of Continuing Medical Education.